Advance Praise for
The Canyon Ranch Guide to Men's Health

"I think the world of Dr. Brewer. His great work will continue to help and encourage many people."

> —**Tommy Lasorda,** Former Los Angeles Dodgers Manager
> Member of National Baseball Hall of Fame

"In this book, Dr. Brewer brilliantly lights the path to optimal health. Whether you are 18 or 80 or anywhere in between, this is a must read for every man!"

> —**Mel Zuckerman,** Co-Founder Canyon Ranch Resort & Spa

"*The Canyon Ranch Guide to Men's Health* is remarkable on every level. This is truly the definitive men's handbook for better health, fitness, and 'quality of life' no matter what your age. Having been around sports and elite athletes for decades, I was still blown away by the information and insights it contains. Thanks, Dr. Brewer!"

> —**Bill Macatee,** CBS Sports

"I loved the book! A great, easy to understand guide for us guys. Good health is the foundation for everything in our lives. Dr. Brewer's book is a terrific outline for understanding good health and how to sustain it over a lifetime."

> —**Don Knauss,** Former Chairman & CEO of the Clorox Co.
> Director on the Boards of The Kellogg Co., McKesson Co., and the Target Co.

The
Canyon Ranch Guide to Men's Health

The

Canyon Ranch Guide to Men's Health

A DOCTOR'S PRESCRIPTION FOR MALE WELLNESS

Stephen C. Brewer, MD, ABFM

Medical Director, Canyon Ranch in Tucson

SelectBooks, Inc.
New York

This edition published by SelectBooks, Inc.
For information address SelectBooks, Inc., New York, New York.

First Edition

ISBN 978-1-59079-362-6

Library of Congress Cataloging-in-Publication Data
Names: Brewer, Stephen C., 1952- author.
Title: The Canyon Ranch guide to men's health : a doctor's prescription for
  male wellness / Stephen C. Brewer.
Description: First edition. | New York, New York : SelectBooks, Inc., 2016.
|
  Includes index.
Identifiers: LCCN 2015026737 | ISBN 9781590793626 (hardbound book : alk.
  paper)
Subjects: LCSH: Men--Health and hygiene. | Heart--Diseases. | Medicine and
  psychology. | Nutrition. | Exercise.
Classification: LCC RA777.8 .B75 2016 | DDC 613/.04234--dc23 LC record
available at http://lccn.loc.gov/2015026737

Book design by Janice Benight

Manufactured in the United States of America
10 9 8 7 6 5 4 3 2 1

I would like to dedicate this book to my deceased father, Robert J. Brewer, DVM. He was by far the most influential male figure in my life. I am so proud of his service to our country in WWII, in which he flew into battle over Europe. He gave me a love of sports where I learned that personal health and fitness is important in not only becoming an athlete, but more importantly it is a means of remaining in a state of excellent health. As a country veterinarian he exposed me to the world of medicine. Observing his love and dedication as a medical practitioner, I always knew that someday I would follow his footsteps into the world of medicine.

Contents

Foreword

As we wind down the first fifth of the 21st Century, we are challenged by unprecedented preventable disease and economic burden, as we try to digest the avalanche of evolving basic and clinical science. Today we spend more than 18 percent of our gross domestic product on health care. This is a misconception, for most of our expenditures are on "sick care." Seventy-five percent of our expenses are to treat chronic diseases, most of which are preventable and are attributable to our poor health behaviors.

As political parties argue over health-care issues and who pays, the disease and economic burden continues to increase. Irrespective of which political party is in power or which party prevails on any given health issue, what we do know is that our disease and economic burden will continue to increase until the public becomes engaged in the daily pursuit of optimal health and wellness.

My colleague and friend, Dr. Stephen Brewer, has done a huge public service by authoring *The Canyon Ranch Guide to Men's Health*. This book is truly a prescription for health. We now know that men and women's health have certain overlapping similarities, yet they are distinctly different, beginning with the XX and XY chromosomes.

For many years we have assumed that the approach to prevention and clinical care is the same for both sexes. In fact, much of the research that we based our clinical approaches on is flawed because it is based on studies predominately involving middle-aged men. From pharmacologic testing, heart disease, endocrine disorders, and many other areas, it is now clear that male and female health issues are distinctly unique, not only by gender but also through the respective life cycles.

Dr. Brewer has provided us with an easy to understand explanation of the variables in the male life cycle that contribute to optimizing your health. This book not only addresses the common health issues of men, which includes sexual and heart health, but also looks at the psychosocial issues that arise during the different stages of men's lives.

This book comes at a critical juncture in our nation's debate about health care, for it contains the essential information needed to decrease our disease and economic burden and begin to control health-care costs while improving the quality and quantity of life.

This should be recommended reading not only to all men but also all females, since they make the majority of health-care decisions in any family.

—RICHARD H. CARMONA, M.D., MPH, FACS
17th Surgeon General of the United States
Vice Chairman, Canyon Ranch

Preface

Do you have a Y chromosome? If the answer is yes, this book is for you.* In my 35-plus years as a medical doctor, I've seen a clear pattern regarding what motivates my male patients to visit my office. Mostly, it's fear—or acute trauma. Guys will make an appointment if they have a severe laceration or other injury. Up until that point, and sometimes beyond, they'll live with a lot of discomfort.

I'm not going to tell you that you need an appointment for every little thing. Actually, I believe the opposite. This is a do-it-almost-by-yourself guide to making you as healthy as you can be. There are a few things that you really do need to do—and you probably already know what they are. And if you want to read more about them, I present the details.

Here's the quick list:

1. If you smoke, at all, stop.

2. Exercise moderately.

3. Eat moderately, and trade most of the red meat in your diet for plants.

4. Sleep better.

5. If you're going to drink alcohol, make it occasional.

6. Exercise your brain.

---

*If no, you probably know someone who does, so it's for you, too.

7. Stretch your boundaries without breaking them.

8. Know the risk factors for the major chronic diseases and eliminate them.

9. Find a doctor who knows at least as much about prevention as treatment.

10. Don't quit exercising because you can't compete with the 20-year-olds.

If you want the details, jump on in. It doesn't matter what order you read this book in, by the way. Start with your age group, use the index for your area of complaint or concern (yes, there's an entire section on sexual function), or go ahead and start on page one of the Introduction.

This book is based on science, but I will use stories to illustrate my points, and the details and advice herein are drawn from my many years in medical practice (not folk medicine—complementary therapies are often valid, but this is Western empirical science).

When I decided it was time to start working on a new book, I thought about several topics on which I could write. My first thought was to write a second book on peak performance (I co-authored the book *The Everest Principle: How to Achieve the Summit of Your Life*). I love this topic. It's about going beyond disease prevention by finding ways to optimize your health. Another topic that has fascinated me for years has been the pain syndrome fibromyalgia.* Compared to most physicians, I feel I have a good handle on effectively treating this difficult syndrome, and I credit my success to using alternative therapies, specifically acupuncture.

---

* Fibromyalgia is a syndrome that affects women eight times more commonly than men. The symptoms associated with it include diffuse muscle pain, sleep disturbance, and fatigue. The etiology of this syndrome is quite complex. It deals with abnormal pain interpretation and is often associated with emotional trauma.

As fate would have it, I was asked to give a lecture on men's health at Canyon Ranch. As I studied and read about men's health for this lecture, I realized that nearly everything I read on the subject I had either experienced personally or had witnessed during my years of practicing medicine. With this revelation I decided to turn my attention to writing this book on men's health.

I am on the cusp of what numerically could be defined as old age. I think back to when my father was my age, and he looked and appeared to be an old man. I feel I am far from that state of health. Maintaining excellent health has always been an integral part of my life. Almost every day I step out of bed glad, but certainly not elated, to embark on some form of exercise. I perform one of the following: cycle 10 miles, run 3 1/2 miles, or swim 1,000 meters.

I also continue to work on improving my diet and focusing on new techniques to increase my mental clarity and awareness. Through my personal quest to enhance and maintain good health, plus more than thirty years of practicing medicine, I know I have a lot to offer in helping men achieve optimal health.

Acknowledgments

I first want to acknowledge my daughter, Elizabeth, who has been much more than a daughter. She has been a friend and an excellent critic when I needed one. I must recognize my sister, Deborah Brewer, RN, who throughout my life has been my closest personal support. With her experience of over forty years as a practicing nurse, the last seventeen years as a surgical nurse at Mayo Clinic, she has given me a lifelong excitement to practice medicine. I must recognize the many hours of encouragement and advice from Sarah Blexrud. She was the first to read my rough draft of this book and with her editorial eye assured me that what I had written was a publishable book. In addition I want to thank her for restructuring the book to make it into a more readable text.

I would to thank the physicians in the Canyon Ranch medical department for imparting their wisdom in specific areas of this book, most notably Param Dedhia, MD, through his expertise in Sleep Medicine.

I want to acknowledge the nutrition, exercise physiology, and behavioral health departments at Canyon Ranch. They have taught me so much over the years working with them.

I could not have written this book without the backing of Canyon Ranch, especially with the executive help from Morey Brown. I must acknowledge the founders of Canyon Ranch, Mel and Enid Zuckerman and Jerry Cohen, for believing and supporting me through the past twelve years as a medical director at Canyon Ranch. I would like to acknowledge the inspiration I received from being able to work with the former Surgeon General of the U.S., Richard Carmona, MD. I would like to acknowledge the Canyon Ranch photographers, Dennis Farris and Daniel Snyder, who did great work with the photos used in this book.

Finally, I want to express a special thanks to:

My agent, Bill Gladstone

My publishers, Kenzi and Kenichi Sugihara

My editor, Nancy Sugihara

Where Are You Now, and Where Can You Be?

Introduction
Why I Chose Medicine

It was the middle of January in Ohio, and the temperature outside was ten degrees below zero. I was fifteen years old. My oldest sister was in her first year of nursing school, and I was in the process of trying to figure out what I wanted to do for my own career. It was during the weekend, and my dad received a call from a farmer who said he had a cow that was unable to deliver her calf. The cow had been straining for more than a day and the farmer had tried everything he knew but could not birth that calf.

My dad was one of the last of his kind—a country veterinarian in solo practice. He answered his phone twenty-four hours a day. This weekend was typical of most of our weekends. Dad would receive a call from a desperate farmer who needed his help, and when the farmer called, it meant there was real trouble. Farmers made little money so they did everything in their power first before they gave in and called a veterinarian to come out to help them. They would pull and yank at a calf in an attempt to try to deliver it. My dad had a series of cartoon pictures hanging on the wall in his office that depicted a set of sequential pictures of all kinds of broken farm equipment. Finally, the last frame revealed a farmer telling his wife it was time to call the vet to deliver the calf.

Because the weather was so severe, my mom "volunteered" me to accompany my father to help him out. The drive with my father in his vet mobile was always a little uncomfortable. My dad rarely went out of his way to have a conversation with me. We generally just listened to the radio, and I would stare out at the miles of snow-covered farmland as we rolled along to the farmer's home. This day was a little different. My dad broke the typical silence that existed between us by asking me a question. He wanted to know if I had been thinking about what I was going to do in life. I said I was considering going into veterinary medicine. He didn't talk much more on the topic other than to say that there were very few vet schools in this country, and it was becoming more and more difficult to get accepted.

When we arrived at the farm, I did not want to get out of the truck and face the freezing cold. After much self-talk, I dragged myself out of the truck and felt the arctic-like air blast across my face. I grabbed my dad's huge forty-pound medical bag and trudged through the snowdrifts to the barn. In frigid weather like this, the barn gave little respite from the bitterness of the day. I shivered as we walked to the corner of the barn where the exhausted cow lay. Dad was the first to climb over the barn gate in his overalls and huge boots. I followed, carrying his black bag and the big heavy calf puller.

I had done that for years. Carrying his bag was the first job my father assigned me when I began following him on his calls. I often think back and realize how lucky I was to be able to tag along with my father while he worked. I knew everything my father did in his daily trade.

Back in the barn my dad knew this cow was in bad shape. Cows, like horses, do not lie down. They even sleep standing up. When a cow is down, it generally means it is very ill and too exhausted to stand. My dad opened his big black bag and put on his rubber glove, which extended over his whole arm and had a sturdy rubber strap at the end that fit over his head to keep the open end from slipping off. He took out his white plastic spray bottle and sprayed lubricant up and down his entire rubber glove. He then put his whole arm up the cow's backside to feel for the calf's legs. Cows, because their legs are so rigid, deliver differently than humans. Human babies emerge headfirst and calves emerge front legs first. Dad groped and twisted his arm and his entire body trying to move the calf around in a better position for delivery. As beads of sweat built up on Dad's forehead, I stood in the corner of the stall shivering.

Dad said this was going to be a rough delivery and wasn't sure we were going to be able to succeed. He asked me to bring over the calf puller. When put together, the calf-puller was a long metal pole that Dad would position behind the cow. He would then reach into the womb of the cow and attach chains to the front hoofs of the baby calf. The chains were then attached to the calf puller, which had a crank. It was not unlike a winch for pulling vehicles out of a ditch. It was my job to turn the crank, and Dad would try to maneuver the calf. I cranked and Dad tried manipulating the calf so we could pull it out. We worked for more than half an hour, pulling and cranking and straining. Despite all our efforts, the calf didn't budge.

My father finally turned to the farmer and said we would have to do a cesarean section in order to deliver the calf. The farmer had to think long and hard about this. It would add thirty-five dollars to his bill. After deep contemplation, he realized economically he would get more money out of this cow if it lived than if he put it on the butcher's block. He told my father to proceed with the cesarean section.

I had no idea how my dad was now going to perform this tiring procedure. I was already exhausted. Because of the size of the cow and due to the fact that there are no operating tables in a barn, the only way one can access the cow's uterus is through the side of the cow. Dad injected a local numbing agent on the side of the cow's abdomen and proceeded to use his scalpel. To enter a cow's abdomen from the side and to get into the uterus is a feat in itself. My dad kept telling me to hold back parts of the cow's internal organs I didn't know existed.

I pulled and strained, as my dad pulled and strained. The cow looked like it was half dead.

During this whole procedure, the only words that came out of my father's mouth, other than yelling at me to hold this organ or pull on this body part, were swear words that would shock a sailor. I have no idea if his gifted cussing was part of the delivery technique, but my father worked through blood and bowel until the body of a calf appeared. He told me to pull on the hooves, and he worked at positioning the rest of the calf's body to come out the side of this cow. As I pulled this calf out, to my wonderment, its eyes opened and I was the first thing it saw. I knelt there panting but my dad never stopped. He kept working on the inside of the cow to stop the bleeding and then began the long process of sewing up the cow's uterus and then the walls of the abdomen.

When we finished, it had easily been two hours since this whole process had started. The side of me facing the cow was drenched in sweat, and my backside was nearly frozen from the frigid outdoor temperature. Finally, after all was done, my dad turned to me as I sat straddling a bale of hay.

He asked me the same question that he had asked me three hours earlier in the truck, "Stephen, what do you want to be when you grow up?"

I didn't hesitate with my answer. "Dad, I want to wear a long white coat, work inside, and see human beings as patients."

For the first time, my dad broke into a wide grin and said, "Smart decision."

As we left the barn I turned around and looked into the pen where my father and I had just spent the last two hours. There in the corner of the pen stood the mother cow licking away at her tail-wagging newborn calf.

My life began in the early 1950s. I was born in the stereotypical 1950s household, where children were to be seen not heard. I was a child of "The Greatest Generation." Dad fought in Europe in World War II, where he was a waist gunner on the B-17 bombers that were named The Flying Fortress. He was one of the lucky ones who returned from the war physically unscathed. He and his whole generation stated that they had saved the world, and in many ways they had. This affected how they lived after the war. They felt entitled in many ways; the world owed them for what they had sacrificed. They felt they needed to party and celebrate, and the idea of eating healthy and staying fit was the last thing on their minds. They were a social generation that enjoyed cocktail parties and club parties. They had saved the world, and now they were going to reap the rewards.

Cocktail parties were exactly that—a lot of food and booze. Whenever my parents threw a party, it seemed like food was everywhere. "Eat, eat, eat" was the unwritten motto. The object was to pile plates high with food and you were expected to ask for seconds, especially if you were a guy. By today's standards the food was far from healthy. It was a lot of beef, fried foods, and piles of potatoes. Upon completion of the evening meal, the standard joke around the dinner table was to ask what was for dinner on the following night. By the time these men were in their thirties, they generally sported large bellies. These mid-abdominal protrusions symbolized wealth and success.

Alcohol was another issue. It was pretty standard for most people to drink. Those individuals who didn't drink were considered the "oddballs." Homes would commonly have objects that would signal when it was five o'clock, because that was the start of "Happy Hour," such as a classic martini-shaped clock that rang at the five o'clock hour. Friends and families would get together and have drinks and eat appetizers consisting of cheese dips and lunchmeats. No one talked about going out for a walk or run. It was not seasonal. Winter, spring, summer, and fall, 5:00 p.m. meant drinks and happy times.

This made an impression on me and on the rest of the baby boomers. We felt that being a successful grownup meant working hard during the day and coming home and consuming several alcoholic drinks and piles of fat-dripping meat. The evening meal would conclude with a large dessert topped off with whipped cream. If we had company, it often ended with an after-dinner drink. This was the end of another wonderful "healthy" evening!

The other major contributor to this ill health was the prevalence of smoking. It felt like everyone in my parent's generation smoked. Everywhere you went, you were surrounded by smoke. Non-smoking areas didn't exist. When I lived in Cincinnati, it wasn't until the early 1990s that the first non-smoking restaurant finally opened up!

During the sixties it was all about the Beatles, Vietnam, drugs, and free love. The sad scenario is that many of those individuals who made the decision to party more, drink more, and now explore the world of drugs often destroyed their bodies. When I studied Chinese medicine, I learned that the human body has many different forms of energy circulating through it. When the body is abused, it can lose a significant amount of that energy. The Chinese believe that many forms of this nourishing energy can be replenished by eating well, restorative rest, acupuncture, herbals, and tai chi.

There is one form of energy called Yuan chi (energy), which means original chi. This is your core chi (energy), and you are born with it. It has a lot to do with our biologic age, and this chi cannot be replenished. Those individuals who abuse their bodies can lose large amounts of this form of chi, and they are the ones who look 60 when they are only 40 (Keith Richards). The booze, the drugs, the smoking, and the poor diets all accelerate the loss of Yuan chi. These men (and women) will look older than their stated age for the rest of their lives. Improving your health will slow down the loss of Yuan chi, but you cannot get back what you have given away.

During the 1960s when everyone was thinking of how much alcohol they could drink or how much dope they could smoke, I was totally into sports. It was my life. I watched every sporting event and tried to compete in anything that my body would allow me to do. The sporting world was very different then compared to now. People had to create their own sporting reality. Before junior high school, the only organized sport available for kids was little league baseball. I met for one practice a week and one game a week. Now kids have the option of participating in a million and one different athletic classes. They start young and are often shuffled into organized day camps.

Sports were everything to me. I tried all sports, but I excelled in football and golf. My whole focus was to play high school football and then go on to play college football. I did well as a running back at a successful high school program. By the end of my junior year in high school, I was living my dream. The high school football team I played on had gone undefeated and was ranked one of the top schools in the state. I had been the leading rusher and scorer on the team. I had even set a school record on the number of yards rushing. I began to receive letters from all the major Midwestern and Eastern colleges. I thought I had died and gone to heaven the day I received my letter from Woody Hayes, the head football coach of The Ohio State University. I thought I was on my way.

As a child of two Ohio State graduates, Saturdays in the fall meant college football. In those days there were only one or two Ohio State games that were shown on TV, which meant we spent the rest of the season sitting or standing around the radio on Saturday afternoons. I would listen to every Ohio State game and scream and cry throughout the whole game. I knew all the Ohio State players. The highlight of every year was a trip to Columbus, Ohio to actually see a game live. My father usually received alumni tickets to one game per year, and we would travel the two hours in our car to watch the game.

It was always full of traditions. We would park the car at my father's secret parking lot and tailgate with all kinds of food. After that we would walk to the basketball arena, which was right next to the football field and listen to The Ohio State marching band put on their pregame show. The last trek was to walk among the 100,000 screaming fans over to the giant horseshoe of The Ohio State football stadium.

When I received a letter at the end of my junior year from the coach of Ohio State, I was on cloud nine. I trained all summer before my senior year of high school, so I could prove that I was worth their interest and ensure a college football scholarship. On the last week of my high school summer conditioning program, a week before summer practice was to begin, I put on an old pair of football cleats to work out in. The old cleats were longer than my newer ones. For some reason, I ended up running with the defensive backs that evening. The main difference in practice between offensive running backs and defensive running backs is that defensive backs do a lot of running backward. Offensive backs only run forward unless they are really bad.

As I was running backward with the defensive backs, with the longer football cleats, the unthinkable happened to me. I caught my cleats in the turf and twisted my knee. I had the most excruciating pain I have ever experienced in my life. It was as if the top part of my leg disconnected from the bottom part of my leg. The whole practice session stopped. Here I was, the star running back of the top team in the state, and every coach was hovering over me. The trainer ran to the local doctor's home and dragged him over to see me on the field. Through the pain I didn't realize that at that moment my football career was over. I tried a few comebacks but the knee never held up.

We didn't have MRIs back then. A diagnosis of my knee injury was made purely on the physical exam by the orthopedic surgeon. I was taken to an orthopedist in the big city of Dayton, Ohio. I was told it was either a strain or a torn cartilage. He eventually operated on me and removed cartilage, which had nothing to do with my knee problem. It wasn't determined until much later that my knee injury was a torn anterior cruciate ligament. At that time they did not know how to surgically repair this injury and it ended most athletic careers.

As painful as that experience was, it taught me so much about myself and, most important, about the delivery of health care. I had been spoiled as a child when it came to health care. Growing up in a small town with my father as the local veterinarian, our family had ties with the local medical establishment. All the dentists, vets, and doctors treated one another's families like they were their own. If I had a medical problem, my dad would simply take me to the back door of the doctor's office and I could be seen without an appointment. If the office was too crowded, the doctor would send me home and stop by my house after work to see me. When my knee was torn up and I had to be seen by an orthopedist, I didn't realize you had to make an appointment and wait three weeks to be seen. This was my first emergence into real health care.

The second major eye-opening experience was the cold approach I received from the specialist. When I saw the orthopedist, he basically told me I couldn't play football again in a very matter of fact tone. He had no idea that my entire life had tragically been turned upside down. I looked at my parents when the doctor left the exam room, and I broke down and wept. All my contacts with health care providers prior to that episode had been personal family friends. I had always received a personalized touch with small talk, and I was accustomed to having a caring health provider each time I was seen.

To this day I have never forgotten that interchange with the orthopedist. For that reason, whenever I see patients, I always try to start my discussion with something humorous or discuss something outside of their present medical problem. This helps to relax them and, most important, it makes them feel that I am interested in them as a person, not just another patient. It can make a huge difference in the care of that patient.

Even though sports have remained a large part of my life, it has not consumed me as it had before. After this accident I realized that academics were to be my focus, not sports. In many ways, that career-ending injuring pushed me towards my lifelong pursuit of medicine.

Everyman—The Story of Frank

Frank is my "Everyman." And one of the reasons I'm sharing his story first is because, among other things, he wasn't happy with his level of sexual function. I've changed his name, but with his permission I'm including his case study in its entirety. It's not a composite. He's a real guy, still out there walking, talking, and living his (much healthier) life. He's 56 years old, but even if you are younger or older than Frank, you could easily have some of the same problems.

Frank came in to see me because he was overweight and out of shape. He had a successful career on the West Coast in the software industry. He was in semi retirement and he wanted to make a major change in his life. Before he turned fifty he often ran and cycled in groups with men in their late twenties and thirties. He had competed in several triathlons and had run in more than one marathon. When I saw him, he was 30 pounds overweight. He exercised rarely because any time he exercised with his usual crowd, he always found himself at the back of the group. He could no longer keep up. He grew short of breath with exercise, causing him to stop intermittently to catch his breath. Finally, he noted that over the course of the previous year, his libido had been slowly fading away.

When I first saw Frank, I ordered a bone density and body composition scan. It displayed a loss of bone density and a high percentage of body fat, especially around his midline. His blood tests indicated that he had low testosterone, elevated cholesterol, and he was pre-diabetic. I obtained a cardiac stress test to give him clearance to begin exercising again. With Frank's shortness of breath and a past history of allergies, we performed a lung function study to examine his lung status. His stress test revealed that his heart was fine but his fitness level was incredibly low and he had exercise-induced asthma. With this information I prescribed an inhaler to be used prior to exercise.

During my initial interview, in trying to assemble a more complete picture, I asked Frank about his sleep. He told me it was terrible and that he was only averaging five hours at night, and when he did sleep it was of poor quality. Knowing this, I advised Frank to have a sleep study. His sleep study showed that he had significant sleep apnea (these are episodes where a person stops breathing during sleep). We immediately started him on a CPAP (continuous positive air pressure) machine to be worn at night to prevent his breathing disturbances.

I sent Frank to a nutritionist to help revamp his diet. In addition, I sent him to our exercise physiologist to give him a more realistic age-appropriate exercise program to "maintain" his health and not one designed to "compete" against the 30-year olds.

I saw Frank back in the office after he spent a week at Canyon Ranch. He was ecstatic and almost manic. He had not felt this great in years. He was able to exercise without becoming short of breath (he was using the inhaler prior to exercising), he was averaging more than seven hours of uninterrupted sleep at night, and he had lost five pounds. But what he was the most excited about was that his libido had returned.

So what had happened to Frank in just one week? Frank, because of his ultra-competiveness, became frustrated trying to keep up with much younger cyclists and runners. Out of this frustration he literally gave up exercising. With less activity, he began to gain weight. He then started to neglect other aspects of his health, which included his food and drink. He continued to eat as much—and sometimes more—as he had when he was running marathons. Since his body was not burning the calories, it was a simple mathematical equation: more calories in than out means added weight. Also, out of boredom he began drinking more alcohol, which is pure added calories. This increased his weight gain even more. With the additional pounds, especially around the midline, more inflammation is produced in the body (this will be discussed in greater detail later in the book). With more inflammation in the body of a person with a history of allergies, he had a high propensity to develop asthma. With the asthma, exercise became more difficult to accomplish. This in turn led to more weight gain.

The other problem that started with his weight gain was obstructive breathing problems during sleep. Poor sleep has multiple consequences, which includes an increased appetite (causing more weight gain) and decreased production of testosterone (the highest production of testosterone is at night; therefore poor sleep can decrease testosterone production), leading to a lowered libido. Poor sleep has been shown to be another source for increased inflammation in the body. This in turn can worsen asthma. By addressing all of these issues, Frank was able to lose weight and control his asthma. His sleep was dramatically improved, which helped his breathing and increased his ability to exercise again. Finally, with better sleep, his libido was back due to his increased nighttime production of testosterone.

What I love about this case is that in the beginning it seems like a hopeless complicated issue for Frank. However, when broken down, there is a simple logical answer to his poor health and the solution to improving it is simple, attainable, and immediate.

2

It's Time for Men to Take Control of Their Health Care

In my medical career, I have never had an interest in treating only one gender. I became a family physician to treat men, women, and children. However, in my 30 years of practicing medicine, I have spent a lot of time and focus on the health and care of women. The simple reason is that the majority of my patients during the first half of my medical career were women. I estimate that at least 60–70 percent of my patients were women. I never purposely sought out more women. I just put up my shingle and examined whoever walked into the office.

This is not atypical of most general practices. Women generally are more tuned into their bodies than men. They take note of how they feel and address physical and emotional issues much earlier than men do. Through the years it has been my observation that many women seek medical advice when they sense that something is wrong with their bodies. On the other hand, men have the tendency to avoid medical care, even when it is blatantly obvious that something is awry. Men will watch that spot on their arm get bigger and bigger until they finally conclude it just isn't going away. At that point they finally decide to see their doctor. Another common reason men have visited my office over the years is not due to any initiative from themselves but due to a strong encouragement from their wives or significant others.

Since women were the majority of my patients, I have studied women's issues, such as menopause, hormone replacement, and PMS. I also focused on those diseases that were more commonly seen in women than men, such as fibromyalgia and autoimmune diseases like rheumatoid arthritis.

The needs of my female patients led me to study acupuncture and finally to a specialized form of medicine called Integrative Medicine. Women expected their health-care providers to utilize and understand complementary and alternative medicine. My female patients studied alternative medicine and openly asked me, as their medical provider, if I knew about mind-body medicine, vitamins, and acupuncture. I realized if I was going to effectively help and treat these patients, I needed to learn about and possibly practice these forms of therapies. I felt it was important to understand these alternative therapies from a science-based position. I could then critically guide and advise my patients in their use of alternative therapies.

When I first took over as the medical director of Canyon Ranch in Tucson in 2004, my clientele was a much higher proportion of women than men. Over the years the ratio of men to women has slowly changed. My practice is now about fifty/fifty men to women (I no longer see children because Canyon Ranch is an adult wellness center). This increased ratio of male patients has been mostly due to men seeing me for preventative care and not just for acute illnesses. This has been exciting to me.

In my thirty plus years of practicing medicine, I have seen too many middle-aged men become physically handicapped or die of preventable diseases. Too often, my first medical encounter with male patients has been after they have experienced their first heart attack or have already been diagnosed with diabetes. My job at that point is to pick up the pieces and do the best I can to improve their overall health status. After a heart attack the patient may be physically handicapped, unable to work, and have limited endurance. They may experience shortness of breath or have signs of heart failure.

In the case of diabetics, especially those men with poor blood sugar control, they may have one or more of the many complications associated with this disease, including: diabetic neuropathy (nerve damage), which causes numbness and burning in the feet; diabetic retinopathy (damage to the eye retina), which can result in blindness; and diabetic nephropathy (diabetic kidney disease), which can end in kidney failure. Not all but many of these gentlemen could have prevented these complications if they had paid attention to their health.

It's time for men to be more conscious and aware of their health. Men typically think of themselves as being invincible, and they will often fail to seek out medical care until it is too late. In this book I would like to challenge men to be more accountable to their health. They need to be aware of what is right and what is wrong with their bodies. Too many times I see men put on blinders and ignore early signs of disease. I wrote this book to give men the insights and direction they need to have a long and healthy life.

3

The Annual Physical Exam

Do you really need one?

We need to look under the hood of our car every five thousand miles, change the oil, and replace the filter. Now, I am not suggesting we need to have our blood changed after every five thousand miles, but we should look under our own hoods once a year to be sure all our cylinders are running smoothly. The yearly physical is our maintenance check. When I first began practicing medicine in the early 1980s, I thought seeing a doctor for a yearly physical was a waste of time for both the patient and the doctor. I was trained to treat sick people, so why should I spend my time with someone who had no real disease? Why should someone with no real complaints come to my office and take up space that could be used for a sick grandmother or child? I would tell patients there was little need for a routine health check, but they should come and see me when they were ill.

In reality the only time most patients see a doctor is when they are sick. Unfortunately, we now know that by the time a disease produces symptoms, it is often too late to be cured. At that point the objective changes from curing the disease to slowing down its progression. An example of this may be a person who sees a doctor because he has felt fatigued and has had increased urination for several months. If a doctor hears these symptoms, the first thing he or she thinks about is diabetes. At that point the doctor would perform blood tests to see if that patient does, in fact, have diabetes. If the tests confirm diabetes, then a physician will recommend a treatment plan to keep the disease under control but with no real thoughts of a cure. If that same individual had been seeing his doctor annually, the physician could have noticed that his blood sugars were slowly rising, he may have been gaining weight, and his triglycerides were elevating. If these changes were observed on an annual exam, a plan could have been implemented early to put that person on a weight-loss program, improve his diet, and increase his exercise. By making these changes, that person's diabetes may never have developed in the first place.

Physical Exams Can Help Prevent Disease

With all the information that is available about disease prevention, it has become obvious that adults should have routine physicals. I recommend that adults from age 18 to 40 have a physical every other year (more often if they have a chronic illness), and after age 40 they should have one annually. My attitude reversal has been a result of having a clearer understanding on the genesis of many diseases. There are certain risk factors of diseases that if present can increase the chance of developing those diseases. By obtaining routine physicals, a physician can look for those risk factors and attempt to eliminate them.

Unfortunately, men are far less likely than women to come in for a yearly physical. Women since their late teens and early twenties often have seen a doctor for a yearly female exam. Men, on the other hand, feel that they have no reason to see a doctor on a regular basis. They do not need to see a doctor to get a renewal of birth control pills the way women do. Because of this, the idea of obtaining a yearly physical does not pop up on their radar screen. Well, gentlemen, this needs to change. The annual or biannual physical may be one of the first ways to close the mortality gap between men and women. (The life expectancy for a man is 76.4 years and for women is 81.2 years.[1])

Make Lists Prior to Your Visit

Once you have committed to obtaining a yearly exam, you need to make several lists before your physical. These lists will prevent you from forgetting important health issues that need to be discussed during your doctor's visit. The first list contains current health issues that you or your significant other have noticed. Don't ignore the health concerns of your significant other. It is not unusual for those health issues to be crucial in maintaining your health. Your loved one can sometimes see things that you don't recognize or think are important but may well be critical in your health.

The second list needs to contain all the old medical problems that you have experienced. This includes previous hospitalizations, surgeries, and chronic medical conditions, such as high blood pressure, heart disease, or diabetes. Next, list all of your medications, supplements, and vitamins you are taking on a regular and non-regular basis. Don't hide certain supplements because you are afraid your doctor will not approve of them. Drugs, vitamins, and supplements can interact with one another and potentially cause toxicities when taken together.

You should also make a list of all of your potentially harmful habits. You need to be as honest as you can when discussing them. These habits include the usage of tobacco products, alcohol consumption, caffeine consumption, and recreational drug use. Men are notorious for underestimating their usage of these items. This is a good time to have a gut check on these bad habits. Determine if you can cut down or eliminate some of them. Your doctor can give you advice on ways to decrease or get rid of those bad habits that can negatively affect you health.

You will also need a list explaining your family history of diseases. It is important to note if there is a family history of heart disease, strokes, cancers, diabetes, thyroid disease, and autoimmune diseases like rheumatoid arthritis, lupus, and ulcerative colitis. Until we are able to easily interpret our DNA to give us the risk of developing certain diseases, we must rely on a historical model of what diseases have occurred in the family.

Before your visit, write down any problems you may be having with your individual organ systems. That would include your cardiovascular system, your pulmonary (lungs) system, the gastrointestinal system, the genitourinary system, your musculoskeletal system, your nervous system, and questions related to your skin (new moles, darkened moles, rashes, and so on). In that same list, be sure to record how you are feeling emotionally. Do you have bouts of depression? Are you overly anxious? Are you stressed out?

The last list needs to contain information on sleep, exercise, and diet. How long do you sleep? Are you tired during the day? Do you exercise and, if so, what kinds of exercise do you perform (swim, bike, run, and so on)? How frequently do you exercise and for how long? Finally, you need to write down all that you eat. What are your usual meals? How often do you eat? What times of day do you eat? How much do you eat? Do you eat snacks? All of these questions are important for your health.

Vaccinations

Another important health issue that you should discuss with your doctor during your annual visit is whether or not you are up to date with your immunizations. There are contraindications to all the vaccines, such as allergic reactions, that should be discussed with your health-care provider. The following vaccines are the ones most important for adults to receive:

- **Influenza:** This should be obtained yearly. Adults 18 years or older can receive the recombinant influenza vaccine known as RIV (Flublok®). RIV does not contain any egg protein and can be given to age-appropriate persons with an egg allergy of any severity. Healthy, non-pregnant persons aged two to forty-nine years without high-risk medical conditions can receive either intranasal administered live attenuated influenza vaccine (LAIV [FluMist®]) or inactivated influenza vaccine (IIV). Don't fall into the trap that these vaccines cause the flu. You may have some mild upper respiratory symptoms like congestion or a mild headache within 48 hours of the shot but that is about it. And, yes, this vaccine is not always effective. But if one shot has the potential of preventing you from being seriously ill for two weeks, you should have it.

- **Measles-Mumps-Rubella:** Adults born before 1957 are generally considered immune to measles and mumps. Those born in 1957 and after should have documentation of one or more doses of the MMR, unless there is a medical contraindication. People vaccinated before 1979 with either killed mumps vaccine or mumps vaccine of unknown type who are at high risk for mumps infection (for example, people who are working in a health-care facility) should be considered for revaccination with two doses of MMR vaccine.

- **Pneumovac (Pneumonia):** PCV13 should be given to people 50 years of age or older. Adults over the age of 19 who are immunocompromised should also receive it. Those indications need to be discussed with your doctor. For the immunocompromised a single dose of PCV13 should be given at age 19, followed by a single dose of PPSV23 eight weeks later.

- **Varicella (Chickenpox):** All adults who do not have evidence of having had chickenpox, or who were not previously vaccinated, need two doses (the second dose is to be given four to six weeks after the first dose).

- **Shingles:** This is recommended for adults over the age of 60, regardless of whether or not a person has had a previous case of shingles.

- **Tetanus and Diphtheria:** This should be administered every ten years. One time the booster should be substituted with Tdap, which contains the pertussis (whooping cough) vaccine.

- **Haemophilus Influenza Type B (Hib):** One dose of Hib vaccine should be administered to people who do not have a spleen or who have sickle cell disease. If they are planning on having their spleen electively removed because of certain medical reasons, and they have not previously received Hib vaccine, the Hib vaccination needs to be given 14 or more days before the spleen is removed.

- **Polio:** Routine poliovirus vaccination is not necessary in adults residing in the United States. Such individuals are at minimal risk for exposure and most are adequately protected because of vaccination during childhood. However, vaccination is recommended for individuals who are at increased risk for exposure. This includes: travelers to areas or countries where polio is endemic or epidemic, members of communities or

population groups with disease caused by wild polioviruses, unvaccinated adults whose children will receive
OPV, health-care workers who have close contact with
patients who might be excreting wild polioviruses, or
laboratory workers who handle specimens that may
contain polioviruses.

Adults at increased risk who have had a primary
vaccination series with IPV or OPV should receive a single booster dose of IPV. Available data does not indicate
the need for more than a single lifetime booster dose of
IPV. An exception is adults who will be in a polio-ex-
porting or polio-infected country for > four weeks and
received a booster dose > twelve months earlier should
receive an additional dose of IPV or OPV before exiting
that country.

- **Hepatitis:** There are two types of vaccines for two types
  of viruses. For hepatitis A, single-antigen vaccine for-
  mulations should be administered in a two-dose schedule, with the second dose administered at six to twelve
  months later (Havrix) or six to eighteen months later
  (Vaqta). If the combined hepatitis A and hepatitis B vaccine (Twinrix) is used, administer three doses at zero,
  one, and six months.

I strongly suggest obtaining these vaccines. Of all the potential
treatments of infectious diseases, vaccines are the least offensive to the
body. Vaccines use the body's own defense mechanism to specifically
attack the infection. It does this with little side effects. I'm concerned
about the false accusations that argue that children and adults should
not receive vaccines because they cause diseases, such as autism. Now,
especially with social media, these false statements circulate like wild-
fire. Often parents, who come from a very caring place, listen to non-
medical individuals. People without any real scientific basis will say

that vaccines do more harm than good and decide not to vaccinate their children. These children are then unprotected from these diseases. There has been a consequence for this neglect in giving immunizations, as was seen with the outbreak of measles in Disneyland and the outbreak of the mumps with the professional hockey players.

People don't realize how serious many of these diseases can be because they have never seen or experienced them in their lifetime. Since I am over the age of 60, I have witnessed and have personally come down with many of these diseases. I remember having measles when I was five years old. I was covered from head to toe with a rash and had a high fever. I was so ill, and measles was so infectious, that the doctor had to come to my house to see me. When I was in medical school and in my residency-training program, I saw several cases of atypical measles. These individuals were usually college students, they were commonly very ill, and many had to be hospitalized. It began about 15 to 20 years after the measles vaccine was introduced. Atypical measles occurred in individuals who were incompletely immunized against measles. This happened when people were vaccinated by the old killed-virus measles vaccine (which does not provide complete immunity and is no longer available); or they were given attenuated (weakened) live measles vaccine that was inactivated during improper storage.

~~~~~

Over the years I have seen many patients at Canyon Ranch for their routine examination and blood work. The advantage of coming to a health-conscious resort like Canyon Ranch for an annual examination is that patients are able to take the healthy lifestyle changes prescribed to them and immediately begin to incorporate them into their lives. They are able to eat healthy food and have easy access to exercise with all the gyms, fitness classes, and hiking trails. They also are able to learn ways to relax with breathing and meditation classes. By the time they are ready to leave Canyon Ranch, they are already feeling better and have an improved sense of well-being. You may not be able to come to Canyon Ranch for your annual exam, but it is important that you take the prescribed healthy suggestions given to you by your physician and start as soon as possible to make those changes in your life. Don't wait and put it off, otherwise it may never happen. Sometimes it's easier to start with the low hanging fruit. This may be as simple as not eating that bowl of ice cream every night before bedtime or beginning an exercise program with a daily walk. The most important thing is to get started right away while you feel motivated.

It is just as important to find a doctor who is as good at preventing disease as treating disease. One of the first steps in preventive care is obtaining an annual physical to determine the state of your health. To use the auto check-up as a model again, are there any parts that need to be changed, like losing ten pounds before something serious happens? A good preventative physician can perform a yearly physical to look for changes and trends that need to be addressed. Your doctor can help direct you towards a healthier lifestyle in order to prevent disease and promote health.

Your Health at Different Times of Life

Young Men, Ages 18–30

Time is on your side—don't screw it up.

I was talking to my friend David, who was 23 years old, and he shared one of the best statements with me: If your friends are only interesting when you go drinking with them, then you need to question who your friends are. David had just graduated Summa Cum Laude from the school of business at the University of Arizona. In school he had been the head of the University of Arizona running club, and he taught indoor cycling at the university recreational center. We sat down to have coffee together to discuss the life of a twenty-something-year-old man. He had many insights into this age group, and he felt this was an age of exploration. When you look at the great explorers of the past, most were in their twenties when they embarked on their great explorations. The leaders of some of these explorations may have been older, but their troops were composed of adventurous twenty year olds. This age wants to venture out and discover new and interesting things ("To boldly go where no man has gone before!"). Prior to this age, men may have had the desire to explore, but it was not until they were in their twenties that they actually had the means to do so.

Self-Inflicted Health Problems: Sex, Drugs, and Alcohol

Young men in their twenties generally don't have many health issues. They are usually in the best shape they will be in for the rest of their lives. The majority of their health problems are self-induced. This is a result of their underlying urge to explore and to test the waters of life. These explorations may include accidents caused by using illicit substances, operating a motorized device under the influence of drugs or alcohol, or performing risky behaviors, such as unprotected sex.

I have had discussions with psychologists about this particular issue. They have told me it is a symbolic rite of passage for young men to push their limits and "sow their oats." This can be seen with guys who are out drinking all night and then perform some random erratic behavior like driving their cars at high speeds, which can result an injury that has the potential of a lifelong disability or even death. It is beneficial for young men to compete and push their physical limits in a controlled environment like organized sports. However, to test their boundaries to the point where there is a high potential for morbidity or mortality is just plain careless and stupid. Many barriers can be healthy and at the same time give room for exploration.

This is one area where women appear to be more advanced on the evolutionary scale. They will try some risky behaviors but generally do not undertake the amount or level of risky behavior young men do. These behaviors appear to be on the increase. This can be seen with drug use including "designer" drugs (sometimes enabled by permissive parents who have misconceptions about these), particularly when using marijuana with THC levels that are much higher than they were 30 years ago. There is also an increase in unprotected sexual activity. With all these risky behaviors in this age group, it is not surprising that the number one cause of death in young men ages eighteen to thirty is accidents.[2] This may have a lot to do with the sudden increased production of testosterone.

Channel Energy into Sports

This newfound energy and aggressiveness can be directed in a more positive way. Young men need to engage in more physical activities to improve their overall health. After going to football or basketball practice in school, the last thing I wanted to do was go out and run around late at night and potentially get into trouble. I just wanted to come home, watch a little TV, and then do my homework. Positive physical activity does not have to be organized sports. In college my daughter went hiking and mountain climbing with "the boys" every weekend. At the end of the day, after hiking and climbing, these college students would all return physically tired, their smartphones filled with great photos ready to be uploaded to Facebook and Instagram.

It does little good to rant and rave as a parent and tell our sons not to participate in risky behaviors if we can't set positive examples ourselves. Sitting around drinking excessive alcohol, not exercising, and telling tales of the wild things we once did when we were young is hardly the example to give to our young men. We need to support our sons in their exercise programs and participate in regular exercise ourselves. We need to be more aware of the potential impression that can result in the minds of these young men when we exaggerate our supposed exploits.

So what kind of physical exploits do I recommend? Obviously, I'm an advocate for organized sports. Here, under the eyes of a good coach, young men can push their physical limits in a relatively safe space. I realize not everyone can play in high school or college sports, especially as competitive as it has become. However, there are plenty of running, cycling, or hiking groups. If you cannot find a group, then make your own. With everyone's easy access to the Internet, there are websites designated for active groups. One such group is meetup. com. In our community of Tucson, Arizona, one woman had a vision to increase the activity of all ages in a healthy fashion. She started a weekly meetup group in downtown Tucson where walkers and runners could gather and walk or run at their own pace in a loose fashion throughout Tucson's downtown. There is no massive start, so there are no losers, only winners. This weekly event will gather between 400 and 900 participants, depending on the weather.

Finding a Career Path

As young men reach their late twenties, several issues appear. The first issue is that their careers suddenly become more important. Some men have attended college, while others have gone into the workforce directly out of high school. At this age it is important that these men have direction and are on their chosen career paths. This is not to say that later on in life a person cannot change his life or career path. I am a perfect example of that. In my late forties, I changed my career path from being a family physician to teaching and becoming a consultant in a specialized type of medicine called Integrative Medicine. The objective for this age group is to spend time and energy on a particular life path. Young men often struggle at this stage because they are torn between going out with their friends to play versus trying to focus on their careers.

Handling Insecurity

In my coffee talks with David and other men in their twenties, the one aspect of their lives that surprised me to learn about was their high level of insecurity. Until I had talked with to these young men, I had forgotten and obviously suppressed all the insecurities that I had experienced when I was in my twenties. With all the boldness that is seen in this age group, it was surprising to discover how insecure they are. One of the results of these insecurities is that men tend to run in packs. This is simply due to a "safety in numbers" mentality. Unfortunately, with the protection young men feel in a group, there is a tendency for them to be greater risk takers. When this happens, they push their limits and often get themselves into trouble.

I had a conversation with my 24-year-old patient, Mike, who was in his second year of medical school. On the surface he appeared to be confident and ready to take on the world. I asked him if he had any problems with insecurity, and I was taken aback when he openly admitted that he felt deeply insecure about relationships, his future, and his career. He acknowledged that men in their twenties begin to feel insecure when they are breaking their ties with their parents. This group talks a lot about taking on the world, but carrying this out can be frightening. What if they fail? In the past their parents were their safety net. Now that net is being pulled away. This is the core reason for many of their insecurities.

Mike struggled with finding and developing a relationship. In college he never drank much because he was a competitive athlete. After his competitive days were over, he started to drink a lot more alcohol so he would have the courage to talk to girls. I thought back to when I was in my twenties and felt alone in my insecurities. I too turned to alcohol to give me the courage to talk to the opposite sex. It is important for a young man to realize he isn't the only one who feels this way. My patient, Mike, suddenly felt relaxed and appeared to be in a much better space, when I told him it was a common problem of men in their twenties to have self-doubt. He also realized that going out and getting drunk just to have the nerve to talk to a girl was silly.

I think it is important for twenty-year-olds to admit their insecurities and to discuss them among their peers. Giving young men the opportunity to discuss their anxieties prevents them from burying those feelings and never really addressing them. They don't necessarily need a professional; simply sitting down with a friend or an older gentleman over coffee and being open about your insecurities may be just what the doctor ordered. Realizing you aren't the only one who is having this problem is often the start in relieving the anxiety and fear that is associated with it.

Watch Out for Concussions

I cannot talk about men in this age group without discussing concussions. It is a significant health issue during these years. As I was writing this book, the legal case involving head traumas in the NFL was being decided. This is a significant medical problem. In speaking with older gentlemen who played football, they often talk about the players who experienced concussions and had to be carried off the field. After sitting out a few plays, these players would usually return to the playing field. These old storytellers can't understand what all the fuss is about these days with concussions, and they believe that the present-day ballplayers are a bunch of overprotective prima donnas. They couldn't be any further from the truth. This is one of the most serious problems associated with athletics outside of spinal cord injures or undiagnosed cardiac conditions.

There are a lot of misconceptions about concussions. The general public's perception of a concussion is that people are hit in the head and knocked out. When they regain consciousness, they are nauseated and often vomit. They may feel bad for a day, but then all is well. In actuality, when a concussion occurs there is an injury to the brain from a direct blow to the head, face, or neck. It can also result from a blow anywhere to the body, which transmits that force to the head. Typically, there is a short-term impairment of neurological function that generally but not always resolves spontaneously. With a concussion there is no actual structural change to the brain. The misnomer about a concussion is the belief that a person must have a loss of consciousness. This is not true. There may or may not be a loss of consciousness with the injury.

Initial problems associated with a concussion include nausea, vomiting, headache, and confusion, with possible short-term memory loss. A person may have persistent and sometimes progressive problems following this type of injury. This is called post-concussion syndrome. The symptoms associated with this complex include: persistent headache, dizziness, and neuropsychiatric symptoms, such as depression and cognitive impairment. This occurs more often than people first thought. It is seen in more than 30 percent of people who suffered a mild to moderate brain trauma. (Some studies have revealed post concussion syndrome to be as high as 80 percent.) It is important to note that post concussive syndrome is not always correlated with the severity of the initial brain injury.[3]

Football is not the only sport that sustains concussions. It can be seen with other sports, such as hockey, soccer, and lacrosse. We see concussions when boys are being boys. As was discussed previously, boys love to push their limits, which can result in head injuries. Many of these accidents occur when young men are trying to impress girls by doing antics, such as handstands or trying to tight rope. Another situation we don't talk that much about are the concussions suffered by soldiers in war zones. The very nature of being a soldier increases the risk of sustaining a concussion. In a study of 2,525 army infantry soldiers in Iraq, 5 percent reported being injured with loss of consciousness and 10 percent reported being injured with an associated altered state of consciousness.[4]

In some individuals, especially those who have had more than one concussion, there is the potential to develop a progressive neurologic dementia. This is called chronic traumatic encephalopathy. It has some of the same pathologic changes to the brain as seen in other neurodegenerative diseases like Alzheimer's. These changes include protein deposits in the brain tissue called tau protein. You can see this with men who have played professional sports and have developed severe memory lapses. There is an excellent documentary film about this called *Head Games,* and PBS had a special related to it on *Frontline.* Both of these programs are well worth watching.

Because of my love for football, I have internally struggled with this problem. We know that football has become an increasingly violent sport despite all the new rules trying to prevent it. When I played football, I was 180 pounds and six feet tall. I ran the 40-yard dash in 4.8 seconds. At that time, with those numbers, I was a highly recruited running back by all the major college programs. Today with those numbers I couldn't make it as the water boy. Ballplayers now are well over 200 pounds and many times over 300 pounds. Practically all the players run the 40-yard dash under 4.8 seconds! If you take the Newtonian formula of mass x velocity = momentum, you suddenly realize the incredible amount of impact that can occur with every play.

Because the players are getting faster and bigger in all sports, I fear there will be more head injuries in the future. As much as I love sports, especially football, if I had a son today, I would not encourage him to be involved in contact sports. This is something that every parent and individual needs to grapple with in the future. With the potential long-term consequence that can occur as a result of head injuries, the decision to participate in contact sports should not be taken lightly.

Recently when I was giving a lecture on dementias at Canyon Ranch, I relayed my concerns about brain injuries in contact sports and made the statement that unless the powers to be can make the sport much safer by changing the game and the equipment, the future of football over the next ten years is up in the air. An angry man in his late 60s stood up and said I didn't know what I was talking about and that football was here to stay. He said there is too much money involved and they could never get rid of America's greatest pastime. It was interesting that the women in the audience were in almost total agreement with what I said. In the future I feel it may be the moms who will ultimately make the decision if their sons will participate in contact sports, especially football.

The brain is arguably the most important organ in the body. It makes us who we are as individuals. As I get older the idea of losing my mental faculties earlier than what will occur in normal aging is frightening to me. We can strain a muscle, and with a little time and patience that strained muscle will eventually heal. If we injure the brain, it may heal or it could result in a progressive form of dementia.

This age of young men have the energy and zeal to take on the world at high speed. The energy they posses needs be used in a positive not a destructive fashion. It should be used to spearhead new innovative projects at work, take on jobs to improve the community, and help out with the many special needs that arise in every family. Men need to utilize this wonderful given energy in healthy ways and avoid using that excess energy towards a potentially downward destructive path.

5

Middle-Aged Men, Ages 31–50

It's not too late to change your lifestyle.

At this age, men are typically in overdrive with their careers. This is when most men are trying to "make their mark" in life. Because a man's attention at this age is on his career, his focus is often not on his health. Men will ease off or stop their exercise programs altogether. They feel they are too busy to work out. Instead of exercising after work, they often end up at happy hour "business meetings." I have heard this for years from this age group. They insist they don't have time to care for themselves. If these gentlemen would take 30–60 minutes a day to exercise, they would have more energy during the day, be more focused, and generally perform better in their daily jobs.

There is no question that finding the time to maintain a healthy lifestyle is difficult. When I was this age, I tried to exercise four days a week, but it would often drift down to two days a week. This would occur when I was on call at the hospital, when I was swamped at the office (especially during flu season), or when daddy duties called. These were the facts of life. Despite this, unless I was injured, I did not stop exercising. It has been my best drug for maintaining and feeling healthy.

Diet and Exercise

It is important for men to exercise regularly and maintain a healthy diet. Unfortunately, this isn't always the case. Guys will get up in the morning, drive through Starbucks for a cup of Joe, and add on a sweet roll. Lunch is often eating on the run by grabbing a quick burger or eating a stacked-high salami sandwich from the local deli. Because they are working long hours, men often get home late, have two drinks, eat a huge dinner, then fall asleep in that big easy chair watching TV. This is a cycle that has to be broken.

The business happy hour is another concern. Over the years I have often heard that these gentlemen are unable to exercise after work because they conduct a lot of their business over cocktails at that time. If someone is a drinker, no matter how much that person thinks he can carry on business as usual, he generally does not get much accomplished. I am not saying a person can't have an occasional drink. What I am concerned about is repeated and excessive use of alcohol. The sober businessperson will make clearer and better decisions than someone who is under the influence of alcohol.

There is a classic true story related to this issue. It involved two famous actors in their era, Ronald Reagan and Errol Flynn ("the George Clooney" of his time). The two made a movie together. During the production of the movie, Errol Flynn would party and drink almost every night after work. He tried to encourage his costar, Ronald Reagan, to go out with him, but Ronny repeatedly declined. Ronny instead stayed home at night and spent quiet evenings studying his lines.

Because of Flynn's late nights of corralling, he continually slowed down the making of the film. He often arrived late to the set and couldn't remember his lines. At one point the producers considered cancelling the project because of this disruptive behavior. Ronald Regan, on the other hand, was always on the set on time and ready to go to work. Following the making of this movie, Errol Flynn spent the rest of his life in ill health and developed heart disease and liver failure. He died at the early age of fifty. Ronald Reagan had a very different future. He became the fortieth president of the United States and he lived to the ripe old age of 93.

What Motivates Middle-Aged Men to Get Healthy?

A common theme that often brings middle-aged male patients in to see me is the recent loss of someone they know. That person could be a close friend, a relative, or a well-known public figure. When Tim Russert of NBC's *Meet the Press* suddenly died of a heart attack, my waiting room was filled with overweight middle-aged men. These men typically worked 50 or 60 hours a week, overate unhealthy food, drank too much alcohol, didn't exercise, were overstressed, and many were still smoking. It is sad that it takes this kind of loss for men to realize they need to consider making changes in their lifestyle. If a man does come in to see me after a loss, I know I only have a small window of opportunity to address his unhealthy living. It is important to use this time effectively, because these individuals will soon get back on the treadmill of life and return to their unhealthy ways.

When a man comes into my office after witnessing the loss of someone close to him, I focus on improving his unhealthy lifestyle. To accomplish this task, I often have to change the man's perspective on how he views what it means to have fun. I see this as the biggest barrier to a healthy lifestyle for men. For years what many men feel is a fun time and what "everyone else did" may simply not be a healthy choice, such as partying, drinking, and staying up late at night with friends for years. Also coming home after work, opening and drinking a whole bottle of wine, grilling a huge steak, eating a large bowl of ice cream, and then finally falling asleep in the big easy chair in front of the TV is not the path to take if you are planning on hanging around in a healthy state for any length of time.

When I see these gentlemen in my office, I ask them to point out the healthy choices they are making in their lives and then give them positive feedback for accomplishing these choices. After that discussion I learn about all the poor lifestyle choices they are making. This isn't hard—most of my patients will easily volunteer their bad habits. They know what is good for them and what isn't. It is far from rocket science to know that not exercising, overeating, not sleeping, and being overstressed is not a good way to live your life. Most of my patients laugh at the simplicity of the answer.

Changing Your Lifestyle

When my patients consider correcting their bad habits, their biggest fear is that they will have nothing to do for fun. Our society has the misconception that the only good things in life are the bad things in life (What happens in Vegas stays in Vegas!). This thought is pervasive throughout our lives. This subject must be discussed; otherwise, these men will slowly slip back into an unhealthy lifestyle. I often ask my patients to write down healthy fun things they can do. The transition from unhealthy lifestyle choices to healthy lifestyle choices does not take place overnight. Men have the tendency to make the conversion slowly. Once the inertia starts flowing, and they realize how much better they feel by engaging in healthy lifestyles, the closer they become to accomplishing this goal.

To help me determine the level of motivation that a patient has in making healthy lifestyle changes, I use a simple assessment:

- Is this person trying to make changes out of fear?
- Is this person on this path because he was told to make changes in his life?
- Is he ready to improve his lifestyle because he wanted to do it for himself?

If a person answers yes to one of the first two questions, then his success rate in making lifestyle changes will not be as high as the person who answers yes to the last question. This helps direct me on how persuasive I need to be with my patients in directing them to a healthier life.

One of the best ways I have found to convince gentlemen to change their lives is through education. Men prefer black and white reasoning, not necessarily what feels right to them. Most men need to understand what adverse physiologic changes have already occurred in their bodies from poor lifestyle habits. They also need to know the likelihood of further adverse changes if they continue with their unhealthy lifestyle. My experience has taught me that in motivating men it is important to point out the negatives effects of unhealthy living but not to dwell on them.

I find it interesting how people try to motivate others. As I was growing up, motivation was based solely on a negative feedback system. My parents, teachers, and coaches constantly told me how to act and what to do. If I didn't do the right thing, I was yelled at and reprimanded. When I went to medical school, it was a newer school with a young, innovative faculty. Their focus on motivating patients to become healthier was conducted with a positive feedback technique. They often discussed how we could improve things, and whenever we did something right, we were rewarded in some way. Through my years of practicing medicine, the majority of my patients—especially my male patients—have needed a little of both. Patients need to know what the potential consequences will be if they do not improve their lifestyles. This is what stops them in their tracks and gets their attention. On the other hand, positive feedback motivates them as they move towards a healthier lifestyle.

The education starts with knowing one's baseline health. In other words, where is a person starting? This begins with obtaining a good history and physical exam, along with baseline blood studies (see chapter 3: The Annual Physical Exam). With this information, a physician can determine if a person already has an underlying disease state or is on the verge of an illness. The doctor can also assess if a person is at a higher risk of developing a future illness. By using a positive approach, the practitioner can explain how much better a patient can feel by improving his lifestyle.

It is not uncommon for men to have to mull over the information I have given them before they can make any changes. After men listen to what I have to say, they often have to spend time in their "caves" thinking about what they should do. After a period of contemplation, they often return to tell me that they are now infused with the energy to change their lives.

I have had a great advantage working at Canyon Ranch during the last 11 years. The patients I see there are generally more motivated compared to how my patients were in private practice. To make the expense to come to Canyon Ranch, to carve out the time in their busy schedule, and finally to use their vacation time to visit a wellness community usually means they are already motivated to change.

There are some men who need an "in the face" direct approach to their health. The direct approach can be effective if a physician has first earned the man's trust. This is accomplished through a good doctor/patient relationship. Over the years I have found I am generally more direct with men than women. For the appropriate gentleman, I will bluntly tell him he needs to quit smoking and excessive drinking because it is killing him. If a man has been around a lot of coaches during his lifetime, then a direct approach is often effective in helping him improve his lifestyle. Men will listen to people they respect, and accept a blunter approach.

As important as it is to have the motivation to start a healthy lifestyle, it is just as important to have the mindset to maintain a healthy lifestyle. This is usually more difficult to accomplish than making the decision to change. As I tell my patients, the pathway to healthy living is a "way of life." It's not an occasional thought. I get up at 5:00 a.m., put on my running shoes, and take off on the running path because it is "my way of life." No, I don't always jump out of bed excited to exercise. But it is what I do, because I want to be healthy and live as long as possible. I finish my ride or biking and then eat my berries (great antioxidants). At lunch I eat my healthy lunch, which I packed myself, and then go home and eat a healthy dinner. I am in bed early so I can get at least seven hours of sleep. I do this because it is "my way of life." By repeating this kind of pattern, it can become "your way of life."

6

Older Men, Ages 51–65

I can't compete physically with younger men.
Why should I try?

When I think about running as an older man, I like to think about my good friend Jack who called me on the day he turned 60. He had to tell me he had just finished running 20 miles with his group of friends. So many men when they reach milestone ages become depressed and only think about how old they are. Here was Jack who was so excited to tell me that at his *young* age of 60, he had completed this great feat. It was inspirational to me.

I am a little biased toward this age group because I am smack in the middle of it. This is often the beginning of a reflective time in men's lives. I frequently think back on my 30-plus years of practicing medicine and remember when I first started. I loved spending time with the old docs who had practiced for years. After making hospital rounds, I would end up in the doc's lounge, sipping coffee and listening to all the old "war" stories from these docs. I learned so much from their years of experience. Their insights were invaluable to me in the care of my patients. I don't know how I would have managed my first years of practicing medicine without all those hours of coffee talk.

Increase Physical Fitness

Being reflective is nice for a sense of nostalgia. However, it is important during this age not to dwell on the past—this can result in stagnation in your lives. This age is too early to be put out to pasture. There are too many things yet to learn and do.

In this age group, men feel they have the right to benefit from all those long years of hard work. For the first time in their careers, they have time and money to "play." They more frequently go out to eat, vacation, and spend time with their friends and family. It is not unusual for men this age to stop exercising and start eating poorly. They feel they have worked all their lives and they have earned time to rest and fill their bellies with decadent delights. This is the opposite of what they should be doing at this time. Men should be more active in physical fitness roles and more conscious about what they eat. Men at this age will often have substantial downtime and for that reason will burn fewer calories. Men should speed up not slow down at this point in their lives.

As men get older, they feel that strength training is unimportant. They think strength training is for young robust boys slamming at the weights and flexing in front of the mirror. Actually the opposite is true. The older men become, the more they need to strength train. This age group needs to strength train at least two days a week. In this age group it is important to maintain or increase their musculature. When men are younger they can maintain their musculature with little effort, because they have plenty of testosterone. Testosterone is instrumental in building muscle mass. Unfortunately, as men get older, their testosterone decreases, as revealed in a Massachusetts Male Aging Study.[5] With the loss of testosterone, men can lose muscle mass. Strength training is an excellent way to counteract this decline in testosterone. This will help maintain their strength and their balance. The other important reason to strength train and build up muscle is to help reduce body fat. Muscle is the machine that burns calories. The more muscle you have, the more fat you can burn.

This is an interesting time when men are often at the pinnacle of their careers. The difference between this age and previous ages is that instead of trying to get to the top of their chosen field, their focus is staying on top. Men often spend too much time looking over their shoulders at the younger generation, worrying that one of the younger men or women is going to take over their position in the office. Their time should be focused on looking forward to see what else they can accomplish. Instead of trying to stay ahead of the young pack, they need to spend their energy mentoring the next generation, not trying to defeat it.

I don't necessarily feel this is the twilight phase in a man's life and one is just preparing for the inevitable. Many men love to continue to work and push themselves at this time. As part of this age group, I myself find I am working more and exercising more than my junior associates. I work my full-time job at Canyon Ranch as medical director and then at times have worked weekends at urgent care facilities to maintain my medical skills in acute-care medicine.

This is the age in which you have to start getting smart about how you should exercise. You can't simply take off and participate in any exercise that may seem like fun or is challenging. I am a perfect example of that. I have a bad knee that started with my high school football injury and have had three knee surgeries. Most people would say there is no way I should be running at the age of 62. I have been smart about my exercise program, and I only run three miles two times a week on flat, paved surfaces. I have also learned to run by hitting at mid foot instead of the front part of my foot. By running this way, my entire leg receives the total force of hitting the pavement instead of placing too much pressure on my knees or hips. (See Barefoot Running Below.) I also bike or swim at least three days a week instead of running on those days. The swimming and cycling is much better on my knees than running. This has allowed me to run for years beyond what my orthopedic friends thought was possible. If I had a macho attitude that running is all or nothing, I would have quit running and exercising years ago. I often think of my orthopedic friends when I go out for a morning run and watch the sun rise over the Catalina Mountains.

BAREFOOT RUNNING

Barefoot Running is quite popular these days. When you run either literally barefoot, or you wear one of the many barefoot type of shoes, it forces you to hit on your mid-foot. If you continually hit the pavement on either the front or back part of your foot, it places a tremendous amount of force onto the knees and ankles. If you have a preexisting leg injury or arthritis, running and hitting with your mid-foot significantly decreases the force that could potentially make your joints worse.

For that reason, I focus on hitting on my mid-foot, even though I do not actually run in barefoot shoes. I learned this information from our emeritus orthopedic surgeon, Dr. Jon Wang, who visits Canyon Ranch often to educate our staff or educate himself during our monthly educational grand rounds. Jon is the former team physician of the University of Arizona.

Change Your Focus from Competition
to Health Maintenance

After listening to my men's health lecture at Canyon Ranch, Fred came in to see me. He was 53 years old. He had competed in many sports, including distance running, triathlons, trail running, and kickboxing. He always did well. For years he had been able to keep up with the competitive athletes. As he aged, he was having a difficult time staying at the level of the younger competitors, and in his zeal to keep up, he injured his hamstring. His knees were also causing him pain, and he concluded that he was too old to compete anymore. At this point he did what many men do; he stopped exercising altogether. Fred like many guys had the all or nothing attitude. He felt if he couldn't compete with the best, then why should he exercise or work out at all?

When I saw him it had been more than two years since he had seriously worked out. He had gained 30 pounds. His cholesterol was elevated, and his blood pressure had risen to the point that his family physician wanted to place him on medication. I have often seen this occur in this age group with retired professional athletes. When they retire they gain a lot of weight through inactivity, poor diet, and drinking too much alcohol. They feel that once they can no longer compete at a high performance level, they have no desire to work out or exercise. Once again, it's the all or nothing phenomena.

I sat down with Fred and explained how he needed to shift his thinking. Instead of being Mr. Ultra-competitive, he needed to think of exercise as a means of maintaining health, not a mechanism to prove his virility and masculinity. Fred started to work out again when he acknowledged that exercising was no longer a matter of competition but a means of staying healthy and feeling good for years to come. With his resumption of exercise, he began to make changes in his diet and he decreased his alcohol consumption. After six months of this renewed healthy lifestyle, his cholesterol and blood pressure settled into the normal range, and he lost the 30 pounds he had gained from his previous inactivity.

Keep an Eye on Belly Fat

Men in this age group often use the excuse that they are too busy to exercise and make healthy life choices. This is one major difference I have seen between men and women. Women generally spend more time on their health needs than men. Men will argue that they should be using their time for work and not spending it worrying about their health.

My patient Bill was 59 years old when he came to see me at Canyon Ranch for a health evaluation. He had not had a complete physical exam in almost ten years. Over the previous few years, he had been encouraged by his wife to come to Canyon Ranch for a physical examination. Each time she asked him to visit Canyon Ranch, he always had an excuse. Bill's mind changed when his cousin suddenly died of a heart attack at the age of 51.

Bill had occasionally seen his doctor back home and had been diagnosed with having elevated blood pressure and cholesterol. He was started on a blood pressure medicine that caused him to cough. He decided to quit that drug but did not tell his doctor. For his elevated cholesterol, he was placed on a statin. He stopped that medication because it caused him to have severe muscle pains. He was five foot ten and weighed 235 pounds when I saw him. During my history taking, we discussed his exercise program. He was happy to tell me he had a personal trainer and worked out two times a week. His exercise program consisted of working out for an hour with weights.

Bill's physical revealed that his blood pressure was 162/96. We performed a dexa body composition (see box) and found that he was 42 percent body fat and he had 135 pounds of muscle. The goal for a man is to be under 25 percent body fat to decrease his risk of chronic diseases, such as heart disease, diabetes, and cancer. It is important to note that the majority of his fat was in his mid-abdominal region (better known as his belly fat). Here he was 47 percent body fat. We will discuss later how belly fat can produce chemicals that can increase inflammation and blood pressure in the body. Bill needed a lot of work. His blood work showed:

- **Total Cholesterol:** 232 milligrams/deciliter
- **LDL cholesterol** (the bad carrier of cholesterol): 165 milligrams/deciliter
- **Apolipoprotein B** was 115 (the importance of this protein will be discussed in the heart chapter)
- **HDL Cholesterol** (the good carrier of cholesterol): 32 milligrams/deciliter
- **Triglycerides:** 178 milligrams/deciliter
- **Fasting blood sugar:** 114 milligrams/deciliter
- **Hemoglobin A1C** (the test for three month blood sugar control): 6.4 percent
- **C-Reactive Protein** (The measure of inflammation in the body): 4.5

||||||||||||||||||||||||||||||||||||||||||||||||||||||||||||||||||||||||||||||||||||||||||||||||||||||||

DEXA BODY SCAN

We have the luxury at Canyon Ranch of using a dexa body scan. This is the Gold Standard for measuring body composition. One can also get good results utilizing calipers (these are metal pinchers that grab onto body fat in specified areas of the body). With this tool you can obtain a good estimate of your percent of body fat. (If you subtract that total from your total weight then subtract again six pounds for bone weight. That number is a good estimate of your muscle mass.)

||||||||||||||||||||||||||||||||||||||||||||||||||||||||||||||||||||||||||||||||||||||||||||||||||||||||

Between his body fat and blood work—which revealed high cholesterol, blood sugar, and inflammation—Bill was at a very high risk for having a heart attack and/or diabetes. His risk factors for having a heart attack included elevated blood pressure, increased LDL (bad cholesterol), increased apolipoprotein B, low HDL (good cholesterol), elevated blood sugar, and a high C-reactive protein. The C-reactive protein is a nonspecific test for inflammation but it does not tell you what is causing the inflammation. I could not find an obvious source for this increased inflammation, such as a low-grade sinus infection, a dental infection, a bad skin condition, or a cold virus. When I ruled out infectious and autoimmune causes for an elevated CRP, I was left with his belly fat as the probable origin. Belly fat has the potential to produce multiple chemicals, some of which can cause an increased inflammation in the body.

There were certain results that placed Bill at a high risk for developing diabetes. These were a fasting blood sugar between 100 and 125 milligrams/deciliter, above normal HbA1C (< 5.6 % is normal), increased triglycerides (> 150 milligrams/deciliter), low HDL (< 40 mg/dl), an elevated blood pressure (> 140/90) and an enlarged belly.

We immediately went to work on Bill, sending him first to see the exercise physiologist. Because he already had a large muscle mass ready to burn up calories the physiologist focused on increasing his cardiovascular workout, not more weight training. Think of your muscles as the engine to burn up the calories and cardiovascular exercises as the means of actually burning up of the calories. A large engine is capable of burning more calories than a small engine. Bill's problem was he had a great engine to burn up the fuel (calories) but wasn't using it because he was not doing any cardiovascular exercises.

It was important to find a cardiovascular workout that Bill would actually do. He began using our elliptical trainer because he owned one himself that was sitting in his basement collecting dust. We sent him to a nutritionist who placed him on a Mediterranean diet because of its known benefit in decreasing overall mortality, especially cardiovascular disease.[6] The nutritionist determined that Bill had been eating a large quantity of simple carbs instead of complex carbs. This meant no more three scoops of sugar in his iced tea, no more ice cream before bedtime, and no more three glasses of wine with dinner. Eating to lose weight often is no more complex than eating healthy and getting rid of those foods and drinks that 95 percent of us already know are bad for us.

THE MEDITERRANEAN DIET

The Mediterranean Diet consists of:

- Eating primarily plant-based foods, such as fruits and vegetables, whole grains, legumes, and nuts
- Replacing butter with healthy fats, such as olive oil
- Using herbs and spices instead of salt to flavor foods
- Limiting red meat
- Eating fish and poultry at least twice a week

Finally, Bill saw one of our behavioral therapists. He did a little kicking and minor screaming beforehand because he felt there was no reason for him to see a "shrink." After being convinced of the importance of seeing a behavioral therapist, Bill finally relented and went to see someone. Afterward, Bill personally thanked me for insisting that he see the therapist. The behaviorist determined that Bill was much more stressed than anyone realized. He was dealing with the financial issues of two children in college and his third child had just moved back home because he didn't have a job. He was worried about his aging parents, who were showing signs of dementia, and who lived 1,000 miles from him. Finally, he had to fire a long-time employee, because there was a concern he may have been embezzling in his business.

All these stressors were affecting his health and increasing his cortisol levels. This was confirmed by a lab study. The elevated cortisol levels contributed to his weight gain, his high blood pressure, and increasing blood sugars. The mechanism for these elevations is a complex biochemical response that includes insulin resistance. Our behavioral therapist gave Bill tools to help deal with his stressors. One of his tools was a daily routine of meditation. During this meditative time (which was only five to ten minutes twice a day), he was able to disengage from his constant stressors and have time to relax. Bill left Canyon Ranch with a commitment to this new program. Eight months later Bill was 35 pounds lighter, his blood pressure was 135/85, fasting blood sugar was 97, LDL cholesterol was 98, Triglycerides were 108, HDL was 45, and his fasting cortisol was now in the normal range. Bill could not have been happier.

Heart Disease and Cancer

The risk of health problems increases in this age group. This is the time when we pay for the sins of our past. Those individuals who have a history of smoking, are overweight, and have not exercised are at a much higher risk for developing heart disease. The consequences of not addressing the risk factors for diseases earlier in our lives begins to surface during this age group. The longer you wait to address these factors, the more difficult it is to prevent disease.

Cancer is the second most common cause of death in this age group. This is the age when men start obtaining yearly PSAs, because the incidence of prostate cancer increases. Other screenings for cancer begin during this age group as well. You should obtain your first colonoscopy at 50 years old. It should then be repeated every three to ten years, depending on what is found on the colonoscopy and your family history. If you have a strong family history of colon cancer then your first colonoscopy should occur before the age of fifty. The specific time should be discussed with your doctor.

Mentoring Can Keep You Young at Heart

This is a great time to become a mentor to someone younger than you. You have at least fifty years of life experiences under your belt, and it would be a shame not to impart some of that knowledge and experience into some eager young mind. One of the positive aspects of mentoring is that the mentor will often gain as much from the interchange as the person who is being educated. There is a real thrill and joy from imparting new, interesting knowledge to an eager young mind.

I have loved teaching to all levels of higher education, and I have often been a guest lecturer to the undergraduates at the School of Public Health at the University of Arizona. The fun part is going into a classroom of 200 students and wowing them enough to keep them awake for an 8:00 a.m. class. They are so eager to learn, and I love their youth and energy. I especially love the fact that they are convinced they have the capability of changing the world. I feel ten years younger every time I give this lecture.

Teaching medical students and residents is another wonderful group that I have the opportunity to mentor. This usually occurs one-on-one. I will see a patient with a medical student or medical resident, and they will observe my interviewing technique. Between patients, we discuss the medical issues that were presented during the patient visit. Every time I am with these students my mind comes alive. The more I teach, the more I want to teach.

Even though I love working with young students of medicine, my favorite group to lecture to is a well-educated general public. These individuals come to my talks simply to learn. I do a lot of lecturing to the guests at Canyon Ranch. I lecture on many topics, which include men's health, brain health, weight loss, optimal wellness, heart health, integrative medicine, genetics, and preventative medicine. It is not unusual to have a packed house with individuals who are eager to learn.

This is a transition stage in men's lives. Men no longer are considered to be young at this age. This is the time when men start to look in the mirror and realize that the age thing has started. Time is running out for making the kind of healthy lifestyle changes that are needed to potentially slow down the aging process. Despite this, it doesn't mean you should quit and not try to improve your lives. The important thing is that you can still make an impact on how you look and feel by fighting back and making healthy changes in your life. It's amazing how much younger we can look and feel after a 20- to 30-pound weight loss.

Mostly Retired Men, Ages 66–80

Accepting the fact of being older—moving forward

All the baby boomers are now approaching this age, which makes it one of the fastest growing groups. I call it the slow-down age, because they realize they can't do what they used to do. It is the time when men have to acknowledge their chronologic age. They tire more easily and constantly need to remind themselves to exercise.

This can be an emotionally difficult time, because men in this age group see peers with mental deterioration and onsets of dementia. This is the time when they lose friends and loved ones.

The medical problems seen in this age group are the same as in the previous age group, however, the risk of developing those diseases intensifies. Many other non-life-threatening problems increase in frequency in this age group.

Increased Arthritis

Many men at this age begin to suffer from osteoarthritis, which I refer to as "wear and tear" arthritis. Some people are genetically more predisposed than others to acquire this disease. The disease is a loss of articular cartilage (this is the cartilaginous caps on the ends of bones) and usually affects more than one joint. The joints that take the most abuse through the years are the ones that are most commonly affected by this disease. Those susceptible joints are hips, knees, and hands, especially the first metacarpal carpal joint (the joint where the thumb bone connects to the wrist). This joint takes a beating because we are constantly pinching and holding things.

It is important to use good body mechanics to decrease the stress on susceptible joints. For example, I have degenerative changes in my old football-injured knee. I am still able to run because I focus on three major things. The first is when I run I strive to have good posture. By being more upright when I run (like all the famous marathon runners from Kenya), I put less stress on my knees. It is a more vertical directed force onto my knees so that the whole leg takes the impact of the blow to the pavement. One of the best methods I know to teach a person excellent posture is called the Alexander Technique.* It is commonly taught to actors and ballerinas who need to stand up straight and tall on stage for a better performance. In addition to standing up tall, good posture helps prevent back pains that can develop from standing up for prolonged periods of time on stage.

The second thing I do is focus on striking the ground on the mid portion of my foot (this was discussed in the last chapter). Finally, I no longer run hills or trails. I always look for flat terrains that have smooth surfaces. Doing these simple things has extended my running career at least ten years. There will be a time in the future when my running days will end. When that time arrives, I will not be like Fred, who gave up exercising completely; I will change my tactics and swim more, increase my cycling, and even walk with the older gentlemen.

---

* To learn more about the Alexander Technique visit alexandertechnique.com

Watch Your Balance

Maintaining good physical balance should be a priority for this age group. A loss of balance increases the risk for falls. These falls can result in bruising, lacerations, broken bones, and even brain trauma. Beyond the initial bumps and bruising that may occur from a fall, there are many other potential consequences. These include an increased infection risk and blood clots. Infections in the lungs can stem from limitation of chest movement caused by bruised or broken ribs. Skin infections can occur from open wounds sustained from falls. With less ambulation there is more sitting and lying around, which increases the risk of developing blood clots in the legs.

To have good balance, you must maintain or improve your strength. This can be achieved in many ways. An obvious way is through weight training. You don't need to lift weights for two hours five days a week. I am looking for a minimum of 20 minutes, two to three times a week. If you have not lifted weights before, please be sure to have a qualified trainer teach you how to lift. Strength training does not have to be in a weight room; you can also use elastic bands at home. Some simple strength training exercises using elastic bands can be seen on pages 1, 2, and 3 of the photo insert of this book.

There are other non-strength training exercises that you can use to improve balance. The simplest exercise that I do every day is to stand on one foot when I brush my teeth. Try it sometime. Trust me, it isn't so easy. Performing yoga is another excellent way to improve your balance. To see some balance exercises go to pages 4, 5, 6, and 7 of the photo insert.

Learn New Things

This age is a great time to learn or do something you have always wanted to do. This can be anything from traveling to Europe or studying Ancient Egypt to ballroom dancing or learning Italian or going to the local community college and auditing that class you always wanted to take. The most important thing is not to lie down and wait for the inevitable. Get up from that seat in front of the TV. Move and enjoy life.

Vietnam Vets

During a summer vacation to Minnesota, I met Vern. Because of a gathering of family and friends, I wound up spending my first night in Minnesota at the home of Edie and Vern. Their home was located on the north shore of Lake Superior. It was about ten miles north of Duluth, Minnesota. It is full of birch, pine trees, and gigantic boulders. The weather in mid-August was a perfect 70 degrees. This was a far cry from my usual 105 degrees in Tucson, Arizona at that time of year. It was early morning, and I had just finished running along part of the path where the famous Grandma's Marathon is run every year. When I sat down on their back porch, overlooking Lake Superior, to have a cup of coffee, Edie and Vern came out to join me.

I noticed that Vern had Parkinson's disease when we first met. He had all the classic signs—his movements were slow and he had decreased facial expressions. During our conversation, Vern and Edie found out I was writing a book on men's health. Upon hearing this, Vern and Edie proceeded to tell me about Vern's ill health and how all his present maladies were related to Agent Orange. Not only did Vern suffer from Parkinson's but also he had Prostate cancer and non-Hodgkin's lymphoma. As we talked, I remembered my good friend, Jack, who suffered from a very unusual syndrome that caused his salt level to drop very low. Jack also had been exposed to Agent Orange in Vietnam. These gentlemen are two of the many victims of Agent Orange.

Agent Orange has been a significant problem for this generation of men. During the Vietnam War, our country had a difficult time fighting the enemy because they couldn't see the enemy. Vietnam is covered in jungles, so the military had the bright idea of eliminating the protective cover of the jungles. The answer was Agent Orange. When this deadly chemical was sprayed over the jungle, it killed a wide expanse of the vegetation. Unfortunately, the damage from this chemical was not limited to the vegetation. It did much more than clear the jungles. It had severe toxic effects on humans. Those humans were not only the Vietnamese but also the American ground troops who were fighting in the areas where Agent Orange was sprayed. The effects from these chemicals were shocking. The official statement from the Institute of Medicine of the National Academy of Sciences says that there is an association between Agent Orange and some types of cancers.[7]

The victims who came in direct contact with Agent Orange developed acute skin conditions that often turned into tumors. Others attribute their cancers and multiple miscarriages to living in areas sprayed with the herbicide.[8] The massive number of sick Vietnam veterans, especially those who handled Agent Orange, and Vietnamese civilians has all but eliminated any other possible cause. In addition, many Vietnamese have very high quantities of dioxin in their blood. That substance's toxicity is not disputed.

Among the many complications associated with Agent Orange and dioxin are:

- Skin irritation and skin diseases, such as chloracne[9]
- Neurological disorders
- Nerve disorders, including peripheral neuropathy
- Miscarriages in women
- Type II diabetes
- Birth defects, physical deformities, spina bifida
- Cancers: multiple myeloma, respiratory system cancers, Hodgkin's disease, prostate cancer, leukemia

In 1978, the Veterans Administration set up a program to deal with veterans exposed to Agent Orange. The VA claims to have conducted health exams on 315,000 veterans. Because of the difficulties involved in testing for Agent Orange-caused illnesses, the "VA makes a presumption of Agent Orange exposure for Vietnam veterans."[10] These and other veterans who may have been exposed to toxic herbicides are eligible for health care from the VA.

Vets can receive health care and disability compensation for injuries or health problems related to serving in the military, including Agent Orange exposure. The VA also provides medical care for children of Vietnam veterans whose health problems appear to be caused by Agent Orange (numerous Vietnam War veterans have had children with birth defects apparently attributable to the father or mother's exposure to Agent Orange).

The Vietnam War was different from previous American wars because the American public poorly supported it. These soldiers did not receive the hero's welcome that was typically seen with returning soldiers of the past. This, plus the fact that the 1960s and 1970s were also at the peak of the drug culture, resulted in many Vietnam vets turning to drugs to bury their emotional pain. Not only have these vets had to deal with the mental wounds of the war but also many are still dealing with the added burden of drug addiction.

This age group can have a tough time emotionally because for many this is the first time they look and feel their age. This is especially true if they have not taken care of their health in their earlier years. Because this is an older age group, it is important to recognize the limitations that will occur at this age and then learn to circumvent those limits by doing such things as modifying but not stopping exercise programs.

The one great advantage of this age is that it's the first time many men can look forward to doing the things they always wanted to do.

Prior to this phase in life most men have limited time because of work or family commitments. At this age men can start projects knowing they actually have the time to complete them. They can now see things, go places, and visit people they never had the luxury in to do in the past. In many ways this can a rebirth of that great exploratory phase that epitomized the twenty-year-olds.

8

Elder Statesmen, 80-plus Years

Finding an active routine that works for you

The eighty-plus-year-olds have many special needs. Their health may be a daily issue. From the moment they get out of bed in the morning, they are confronted with health issues. Their whole body feels stiff and their joints ache. Bending over to pick up the morning paper can be a chore. This is why I advise all my elderly gentlemen to start off the day with a fifteen-minute stretch. To see some simple morning stretches go to pages 8, 9, 10, and 11 of the photo insert.

In this age group disease often defines who you are. This can occur in any age group, but it is especially true in this one. You can easily be labeled as the heart patient or the cancer patient. Everything you do or say seems to be related to your health.

Family members of this 80-plus group can unknowingly reinforce this attitude, often telling their father or grandfather that they can't do this or they can't do that because it might be bad for their health. Over time these individuals will assimilate this attitude and, before they know it, they become their disease. Falling into this trap keeps them from doing the things they love to do like playing golf or taking their kids and grandkids out for dinner every Sunday night. They can become frail, depressed, and feel helpless in their ability to care for themselves.

When Family Takes Over

I had a patient, George, who was 81 years old. His two daughters and his wife brought him in to see me. He'd had a heart attack nine months preceding his visit, and his family was doing everything for him since his heart attack. He wasn't allowed to drive. They had a home health care nurse visit him every week, and they had him see a dietician who completely changed his diet. He had been eating the same food all his life, and now the family and the dietician were going to radically change everything he ate. He was being driven by one of his daughters to a weekly heart attack survivor's support group meeting. His wife was forcing him to go to bed two hours earlier than he used to go to sleep. He was taken by his other daughter to twice-weekly yoga classes. The family was calling and checking on him daily. Initially, George thought it was nice that so many people were caring for him.

However, after several weeks of this controlled supervision, George's family and friends noticed changes in George that concerned them. He didn't seem to have the energy he used to have. George was becoming quieter in social situations and his alcohol consumption increased significantly. The family was worried about these changes and was sure something was going wrong with him medically.

Prior to seeing me, the family had taken George to see his cardiologist. After a complete evaluation, the cardiologist said that George checked out fine. In fact, the cardiologist felt that George's recovery far exceeded what he would have expected from a man his age. The family was convinced the cardiologist was mistaken. They were sure he had missed something, so they brought George to see me at

Canyon Ranch for a second opinion. I performed an extensive workup on George, and it was clear to me that he had physically recovered from his heart attack. I brought the patient and family in to see me at the end of my evaluation. I explained my findings to everyone. I told them that I concurred with George's cardiologist and felt he was in excellent shape for someone who had suffered a heart attack. I told everyone that I felt the real problem was that George was suffering from a mild depression, stemming not from having the heart attack but from the simple fact that he had lost his identity. In other words, he was now "George the heart patient." This thought was reinforced with the helpless state the family was placing him in. He needed to be George, the joke-telling former attorney, who loved to play golf, watch football, and have coffee twice a week with the boys. He needed to go to the grandkids' soccer games and scream and yell for their goals. He didn't need to be the weak old man who required help every time he turned around. The family sat stunned when I said this. They thought for sure I was going to tell them that George was overdoing it and that he needed to do less. George was the only one in the room smiling when I delivered the news. I received an e-mail from one of George's daughters six months later telling me that the family had initially been upset with me. They begrudgingly relented and decided to take my advice. To their amazement, within a few weeks, their old dad had returned!

Have a Purpose

Another area that needs to be focused on in this age group is having some form of purpose in life. Having purpose in your daily life is important for all ages, but encouraging men in this older age group to find a purpose is almost essential. Everyone needs a reason to get out of bed in the morning and have something to do. The importance of this was pointed out in the book *The Blue Zones* by the *New York*

Times best-selling author Dan Buettner. In this book Mr. Buettner, in conjunction with the National Institute of Aging, looked at four places on this planet where the population has prolonged life spans. There are several similar aspects between these areas. One of the similarities in these zones is that the individuals who live in these zones all seem to have a purpose. It is especially true with their elderly.

Focusing on having a purpose in the elderly seems to be a bigger problem with men than women. Women throughout their life are generally more social and have a lot more activities outside of work and family. When men retire they feel lost, because they haven't spent as much time outside of work engaged in other activities. I try to explain to men of all ages that there is life beyond work. I know there are a lot of men who feel their work *is* their life. In many ways I have felt the same way. However, when I do get involved in outside interests, like helping my daughter or playing golf, I am more relaxed and more pleasant to be around both at work and away from work.

Having a purpose needs to be more than finding something to occupy your time. It needs to be something that has real meaning. This is very important for the elderly during retirement. I see excitement in men who help out at museums as docents. They have studied the historical significance of the displays. They love imparting their knowledge to the individuals who visit the museums.

I see excitement in the eyes of physicians who, during retirement, return to medical clinics and volunteer their time mentoring interns, residents, and students. The amount of practical knowledge that these older docs can teach to these young students can be as important as what they will learn in all their books or journals. I have seen these students sit back in awe when the old professor gives a simple practical answer to what on the surface seemed like a very complex problem. The old doc swells up with personal joy, knowing he has given back some of that knowledge he has gained from all those years of practicing medicine.

Having meaningful purpose in your life can bring happiness, and as *The Blue Zones* points out, it may be an instrumental piece to your longevity.

Your Health by Function

9

Sexual Function

How things work, and when they don't

Is sex considered an exercise? The answer is yes and no. As much as you may feel you are increasing your heart rate, especially during intercourse, studies have shown it rarely gets the heart rate above 130 beats per minute. The amount of work that is utilized during sex is measured by oxygen consumed. This is measured to be three-and-one-half METS. This corresponds to about the same intensity as raking the leaves or doing the foxtrot. It certainly isn't as low as sitting on the couch and eating popcorn. Sex appears to burn five calories per minute, which is equal to walking a round of golf.[11]

Even though sex does not seem to burn many calories, it does seem to improve longevity, according to the Massachusetts Male Aging Study. In this study they examined more than 900 men who were between the ages of 40 and 70 and did not have erectile dysfunction. They divided the men into groups, according to the frequency with which they had sex. Those who had sex one or less times in a month had 45 percent more risk of developing cardiovascular disease than men who had sex two or more times a week.[12] Hurrah for sex!!!

To appreciate and get the most out of sex, it is important to understand the physiology of a man and woman's body during sex

(If you are heterosexual it is important to know the physiology of the women's body as well as the man's body during sex).

Men's Normal Sexual Response

There are four stages of a man's sexual response: excitement, plateau, orgasm, and resolution. The excitement stage is evident in men with the onset of a penile erection. It may develop within ten seconds of stimulation. Blood is diverted from the iliac artery (which is the supplier of blood to the legs) into the area of the penis called the corpora cavernosa. This rerouting of blood also affects the testes and scrotum. The testes increase in size by 50 to 100 percent and the scrotum thickens and tightens. At the same time muscles in the spermatic cords and scrotum draw the testicles close to the body.

The body prepares for an orgasm by increasing the respiratory rate, the heart rate, and blood pressure. During the plateau phase just before orgasm, the penis is engorged to capacity, and further engorgement of the penile corona and glans (the head of the penis) increases the size and the glans becomes darker in color. At this point a clear mucoid fluid emerges from the end of the penis. This is secreted from the cowper's gland. It amounts to two to three drops. With the ejaculatory phase there is contraction from the prostate, the vas deferens, and seminal vesicles. This is then followed by contractions of the urethra, the perineal muscles, and penile base muscles. All of these contractions result in the ejection of the semen.

This is followed by the refractory stage in which no sexual stimulation can cause a response. The length of this stage varies. It is common for it to be longer in older men. Sorry guys, but no matter how hard you try or how much Viagra you may use, you just have to wait until the refractory phase is over before you are capable of starting the process all over again.

Women's Normal Sexual Response

If your sexual partner is female, it is important to know what is taking place in her body during sex. In women with erotic excitement, there are vascular changes within the vagina that produce a clear fluid. This fluid is slippery and has a distinct odor and flavor. It occurs very rapidly, within seconds of arousal. This fluid is slippery for obvious reasons and it neutralizes the vaginal acidity to aid in sperm survival. This fluid can be decreased with low estrogen states, like menopause, with vaginal infections, and if women are taking certain drugs like antihistamines. As a woman continues to be excited, there is a sexual flush across the upper chest, neck, and back in 70 percent of women. The breasts and areola enlarge due to vascular engorgement, And there is often nipple erection at this time. The clitoris enlarges and is more sensitive to touch. The labia majora and minora will swell during excitement. With an orgasm the perineal, bulbocavernosus, and pubococcygeus muscles rhythmically contract.

Normal Physiology of Obtaining an Erection

We looked at the process of the male sexual response. The key to this response is obtaining an erection. For this development to occur, there must be good blood flow into the penis. The increased blood flow starts with the production of the chemical called nitric oxide. Nitric oxide promotes the blood vessel dilation by increasing the production of cyclic GMP, a second messenger. Cyclic GMP directly acts on the blood vessels to dilate and increase blood flow into the penis. The enzyme that produces nitric oxide is nitric oxide synthase. Low levels of this important enzyme are seen in smokers, diabetics, and in testosterone deficiencies. This is why we commonly see erectile dysfunction with these individuals.

Not only is blood flow important to obtain an erection but also an intact nervous system is essential for normal sexual function.

Erections begin when a man thinks about having sex. An impulse is sent down from the brain to the spinal cord region, thoracic spine eleven to lumbar spine two. From there a nervous impulse is sent to redirect blood flow from the iliac arteries that normally supply blood to the legs to the area of the penis called the corpora cavernosa. A man can also obtain an erection if he is stimulated on the penis or genital regions. A reflex will occur from the stimulation through a nerve to the spinal cord region S-2 to S-4 that will in turn send an impulse to the artery to redirect the blood flow. Therefore, any injury or disease to these two regions of the spine can cause erectile dysfunction.

Hormonal Influence in Obtaining an Erection

The beginning of nocturnal erections begins with the testes production of testosterone. There are two major effects of testosterone. The first is that testosterone increases libido, which causes an erection psychologically by sending signals to the spinal area of T-11 to L-2. Testosterone is also necessary in maintaining nitric oxide synthase levels, which as you read earlier dilates blood vessels and increases blood flow to the penis.

Sexual Dysfunction in Men

Unfortunately, life in the bedroom is not always like we see in the movies. The prevalence of sexual dysfunction in adult men is higher than most men would think. One study revealed that 40 percent of men age 40 acknowledged having some form of sexual dysfunction. In men over 69 years old, 67 percent have an inability to maintain an erection for intercourse.

The definition of impotence (also known as erectile dysfunction or ED) is an inability to maintain an erection for more than 75 percent of the time during the duration of a sexual encounter. There are multiple causes of impotence. It can be related to medications, hormonal deficiencies, neurologic diseases, vascular insufficiencies, and psychological causes.

When and how rapid the onset of impotence occurs is important when trying to determine its root cause. For example, having impotence immediately following a urologic procedure like prostate surgery. This is an obvious cause and effect. The other obvious cause and effect is having decreased libido or erectile dysfunction shortly after starting a new medication.

Most men will have an erection during REM sleep (dream sleep) and will often awake with an erection. If erections have been decreasing or not happening at all at night, there is a high likelihood that this is a physiological or organic problem rather than psychological problem. There are some simple tests that you can try at home under the supervision of a urologist to help determine if you are having erections at night. The testing is called a nocturnal penile tumescence testing. It is simply attaching a device to the penis to determine if you obtain an erection during the night. If this test shows the presence of nighttime erections, then there is a higher likelihood of the impotence being a psychological rather than a physical problem. If the test does not show the presence of nighttime erections, then the impotence is often a physical (organic) etiology.

Sexual dysfunction can simply result from aging. This can be a function of multiple causes, including cardiovascular and neurologic changes that can occur with aging. For a man in his fifties, it often takes two to three times as long as a man in his forties to attain an erection. In addition, the other effect of aging is the inability to regain an erection soon after having an orgasm. All is not lost with aging. It usually takes a longer time for an older male to reach orgasm than a younger male. This can be used to a couples' advantage because it can prolong the act of lovemaking before a man has an orgasm.

Causes of Decreased Libido (Sex Drive)

Whenever I see a patient with decreased libido I always go through the following list of causes in order to hopefully find the source. The answer is not always complex. It may be something very simple, like changing or stopping a medication.

- **Medications:** There are several types of medications that are known to commonly decrease libido. Antidepressants are notorious for lowering your sex drive, especially SSRIs (selective serotonin reuptake inhibitors). The first drug in this class was Prozac. Others in this group include Zoloft, Paxil, Celexa, and Lexapro. 5-alpha-reductase inhibitors also appear to directly decrease libido. These medications are used to shrink the prostate, such as Avodart and Proscar, and treat baldness, such as Propecia. These drugs block the conversion of testosterone to dihydrotestosterone. Most people believe that the major male effects, such as libido and increased musculature, are directly due to testosterone, but in reality it is dihydrotestosterone that causes the male effects. By preventing this conversion of testosterone to dihydrotestosterone, those male effects are blocked. The other group of drugs commonly known to decrease libido are pain medications, especially opiates such as oxycontin and hydrocodone. The bottom line is that if you have decreased libido after starting a new medication, examine medication first as the potential cause.

- **Alcoholism (or excessive drinking):** Many think that alcohol is integral part of the lovemaking dance. This is perpetuated by all the movies over the years showing couples consuming several glasses of wine and champagne prior to scooting off to the bedroom. A drink here or there is not a problem. However, when alcohol consumption becomes chronic and excessive, it is one of the more common causes of decreased libido.

- **Illness:** Any kind of generalized illness can decrease your libido, including infections, kidney disease, auto-immune diseases, heart disease, or cancer. If you are suffering from a systemic illness, you are likely in a survival mode, and the idea of sex is usually not the first thing that comes to mind.

- **Testosterone Deficiencies:** There are several potential causes of decreased testosterone production, including the simple aging process of the testes and pituitary disease. The pituitary produces a hormone that travels to the testicles and stimulates them to produce testosterone. If you have a low testosterone level, try to determine if there is a specific cause for the low testosterone. If the decision is made to use testosterone as a therapy, hopefully you have had a long and serious conversation with your doctor about the pros and cons of using testosterone, especially with the newer studies looking at the connection of cardiovascular disease and usage of testosterone.

- **Recreational Drugs:** Many of the recreational drugs that are consumed have been shown to decrease libido.

- **Fatigue:** "Sorry honey, I am too tired tonight," really is a common cause of decreased libido. The body shuts down and goes into survival hibernation mode and the thought of having sex for men (or women) is the last thing on their mind.

- **Depression:** This is so commonly associated with decreased libido that when I am trying to determine if a person is depressed, I often ask about their sex drive. If they have low libido it leads me to think there is a much higher likelihood this person has depression.

- **Fear of Embarrassment:** This can occur with an especially shy individual who is afraid of being embarrassed and humiliated if he is unable to perform sexually.

- **Relationship Problems:** If a couple is having relationship issues outside the bedroom, then more often than not they will bring those issues into the bedroom. At that point the idea of sex is the last thing on their mind.

Causes of Erectile Dysfunction

There are multiple causes of erectile dysfunction. When most men come to see me because they have erectile dysfunction, they simply want to be given a prescription for Viagra and then go on their merry way. In many cases Viagra and Viagra-like drugs have been helpful, but that should never be the first line of treatment. Always check to be sure there are no underlining correctable causes for erectile dysfunction.

The major causes of erectile dysfunction are listed below. You will note that there are some overlaps with the previously discussed causes of loss of libido.

- **Medications:** Antidepressants (the most common are the SSRIs), spironolactone, sympathetic blockers like clonidine, thiazide diuretics, ketoconazole, cimetadine (but not ranitidine or famotidine) can all cause ED. Once again, just like decreased libido, if you start a new medication and shortly afterward you develop erectile dysfunction, it's likely drug-induced erectile dysfunction.

- **Cardiovascular Disease:** Individuals with cardiovascular disease may have decreased circulation to their penis. It is important to note that if you have erectile dysfunction, it may be an early warning sign of underlying cardiovascular disease. If there is vascular disease to the penis causing obstruction of flow, then you can also have vascular disease in other areas of the body, such as the heart. That is why it is not unusual for some of my patients who simply come in for a prescription of Viagra, will instead walk of out of my office with a prescription for a cardiac stress test.

- **Psychological Problems:** Depression and stress. As discussed previously the normal physiologic response to obtain an erection takes place by first having the brain become aroused to have sex, and then it sends a signal down from the brain to the spinal region to stimulate a nerve to redirect blood flow to the penis. Psychological problems, most commonly depression and anxiety, essentially prevents the initial signal from being sent from the brain and therefore blocks the pathway leading to an erection.

- **Neurological Causes:** These include multiple sclerosis, dementia, pelvic trauma, prostate surgery, spinal cord injury, and stroke. A specific non-mechanical injury to nerves of the autonomic nervous system—the part of the nervous system that regulates involuntary actions of the internal organs—can also cause ED. This is most commonly seen in diabetes, especially in those with poor glucose control. Elevated blood sugars can cause injury to the nerves of the autonomic nervous system, and one of the early signs of this injury is retrograde ejaculation. This is an orgasm that goes backward into the bladder instead of out through the end of the penis. This can be the result of damage to the nerve that supplies the muscles that prevent backflow into the bladder, which can be caused by elevated blood sugars.

- **Bicycling:** The pudendal and cavernosal nerves and blood flow from the cavernosal artery to the penis can be affected by prolonged pressure during long bicycle rides. These nerves and artery are located in the seat area of your body. This can result in penile numbness and impotence. For this reason if you cycle for prolonged time periods, be sure to buy a bicycle seat that takes the pressure off that area of your body. An early sign that this may be occurring is numbness in your seat area.

- **Endocrine Disorders:** Testosterone deficiency, thyroid disease (both excessive and underproduction of the thyroid), and diabetes can all cause dysfunction. With diabetes it is felt to be a twofold effect. The first is the vascular and neurologic damage that can occur from the disease. In addition, it has been found that one third of men with Type II diabetes have low testosterone levels.

Benign Prostatic Hypertrophy (BPH)

This is a common disorder that increases in frequency in men over the age of fifty. The first thing you need to know is that it is a non-cancerous condition. When men start having the symptoms of prostate enlargement, one of their fears is that they are having early signs of prostate cancer (which can cause similar symptoms). Benign prostatic hypertrophy (BPH) is a common condition. The overall prevalence of this process increases from 8 percent in men 31–40 years of age, to

40–50 percent in men 51–60 years of age, to more than 80 percent in men 80 years of age and older.[13] The symptoms associated with this disease are increased urination, decreased urinary flow, difficulty in initiating urinary flow, and getting up multiple times at night to urinate. These symptoms typically come on gradually over the years and are related to the fact that the prostate surrounds the urethra (the piping that takes the urine from the bladder out the end of the penis) as it leaves the bladder. The prostate has the tendency to increase in size as men age. It grows in all directions, including inwardly around the urethra, and essentially squeezes off the flow.

When the obstruction is severe enough that you have a difficult time starting urination, or you are getting up more than twice at night to urinate, then it is time to consider a therapeutic intervention. Benign prostatic hypertrophy can be treated several ways, however you must first rule out other disease states that can cause similar symptoms. These include:

- Cancer of the prostate or bladder
- Bladder stones
- Neurogenic bladder (if the nerves to the bladder have been damaged by disease, such as diabetes, or injury)
- Urinary tract infection or a prostatitis
- Stricture in the urethra from trauma or past infection

There are simple tests that your doctor can perform to help rule out some of these more serious urologic problems with similar symptoms as benign prostatic hypertrophy. These tests include: a urinalysis, a urine culture, and a PSA.

If after having these tests and consulting with your doctor, it is determined that you do not have any of the more serious urological problems and the diagnosis is benign prostatic hypertrophy (BPH), consider the following treatments. First, I advise my patients to try behavioral modifications. This includes decreasing caffeine and alcohol consumption; avoid drinking a lot of fluids prior to bedtime and double void (urinate) to empty the bladder more completely. Double voiding is just that—urinate once then try to urinate again. Next, do not use medications that can exacerbate your symptoms or induce urinary retention. These include anticholinergic medications, such as antihistamines (Benadryl is an example) and adrenergic agents, such as decongestants. I can't tell you the number of phone calls I have received through the years from older men who were treating their allergy or cold symptoms with one of the over-the-counter antihistamines or decongestants and suddenly finding out they were having a difficult time trying to urinate.

If symptoms persist or worsen despite making behavioral modifications, I may advise a trial of medication. There are two classes of drugs used for BPH. They are alpha-adrenergic antagonists and 5-alpha-reductase inhibitors. The alpha-adrenergic antagonists work by relaxing smooth muscles in the bladder neck, prostate capsule, and prostatic urethra. There are five long-acting alpha-1-antagonists—terazosin, doxazosin, tamsulosin, alfuzosin and silodosin—that have been approved by the Food and Drug Administration in the United States. The most significant side effect with these drugs is the potential of developing low blood pressure. These drugs were initially developed to treat high blood pressure by relaxing smooth muscles in the walls of the arteries. It was discovered that it also relaxed the muscles around the prostate, which allowed better flow of urine from the bladder. The newer forms of these drugs are more specific for the muscles around the prostate and have less effect on a person's blood pressure.

The other group of medications used to treat BPH is the 5-alpha-reductase inhibitors. There are two 5-alpha-reductase inhibitors approved in the United States: finasteride and dutasteride. The efficacy of these drugs is greater in men with larger prostate volumes than in men with smaller prostate volumes. These drugs work by reducing the size of the prostate gland. You have to take the medication for six to twelve months before the prostate size is sufficiently reduced to improve symptoms. These drugs prevent the conversion of testosterone to dihydrotestosterone in the prostate. The major side effects of these drugs are decreased libido and erectile dysfunction. My first choice for my patients is usually one of the alpha-adrenergic antagonists. They start to work almost immediately, and if you use one of the newer, more selective drugs, there is little hypotension (low blood pressure). The main reasons I don't like the 5-alpha-reductase inhibitors are due to the potential side effects of these drugs and the length of time it takes for the medication to work.

Herbal therapies for BPH are commonly used in Europe. The United States Food and Drug Administration has not approved any herbal therapy for BPH, although many of my patients have tried these treatments. The most commonly used herbal for BPH is saw palmetto. The exact mechanism of action is unknown, and there is little data to support its efficacy. If my patients want to try a natural non-pharmacologic treatment first for BPH, I will give them the option to try saw palmetto. If they benefit from the saw palmetto that is a plus, however, in my personal practice, I have seen mixed results at best.

Prostatitis (Prostate Inflammation)

There are two forms of prostatitis: acute and chronic. This is more common than many people realize. The acute form is a rapid onset, and you can become extremely ill. For many men it may be the sickest they have ever been. The symptoms come on quickly with spiking fevers, chills, severe muscle pain, and a feeling of exhaustion. The urinary tract symptoms include urinary frequency, urgency, and difficulty starting urination. There is often pain at the end of the penis.

As I have told my medical students through the years, male patients with acute prostatitis do not always present with urinary tract symptoms. If a man comes in to see me with a high fever, chills, and feels awful, I always put acute prostatitis close to the top of my list of probable causes. The prostate is usually exquisitely tender during this acute phase. If the prostate is digitally examined during this time, the patient may have to be pulled down from the ceiling. This is a serious illness that must be addressed as soon as possible and treated with antibiotics. This is not the time or place to attempt to gut it out or try some herbal treatment that your friend may suggest. Over the years I have hospitalized more than one man with this condition, especially those men who felt they could "work through it."

Chronic Prostatitis encompasses several different disease states. They are chronic infectious (bacterial) prostatitis, chronic prostatitis/chronic pelvic pain syndrome that is inflammatory, chronic prostatitis/chronic pelvic pain syndrome that is non-inflammatory, and asymptomatic inflammatory prostatitis. These syndromes usually start off as a bacterial prostatitis. Following the acute infection phase, a chronic process may begin that can result in one of the previously stated forms of chronic prostatitis. The interesting aspect of these chronic conditions is that once it is in this chronic state, only about 10 percent show positive cultures for infection. The symptoms with chronic prostatitis can be pain in the floor of the pelvis, lower back, the penis, the testicles, or the abdomen. There is often discomfort with urination and ejaculation.

This can be a difficult disease to treat. The treatments are not always successful and the patient can be left with chronic pain and discomfort, which can lead to fatigue and depressive episodes. The treatment begins after a urinalysis and culture have been performed. (It is important to rule out a potentially treatable infection.) Even if there is a negative culture, the majority of doctors will still initially place the patient on antibiotics, usually one of the fluoroquinolones like ciprofloxacin. If there are significant symptoms, a trial of an alpha-blocker and sometimes a 5-alpha-reductase inhibitor (discussed earlier with BPH) can be tried. I generally do not use the 5-alpha-reductase inhibitors for my younger male patients for the reasons stated earlier in this chapter.

For those who have chronic inflammatory, noninfectious chronic prostatitis, I suggest a trial of anti-inflammatory agents, like ibuprofen. Often I have seen dramatic improvement of the pain and discomfort in those patients who are suffering from flare-ups of this form of chronic prostatitis.

Peyronie's Disease

Another cause of erectile dysfunction, which is not often talked about, is Peyronie's disease. This disease is a variety of deformities of the penis that can occur when the penis is erect. With this disease there is scarring of the tunica albuginea, the tough connective tissue layer that surrounds the penis. The scarring of this tissue will cause deformities in the curvature of the penis. This results in narrowing and shortening in the tissue that ultimately causes a buckling of the penis during an erection. This disease is more common than originally thought; studies have shown it to be in 3 to 9 percent of men.[14] It can occur in teenagers but the incidence increases with age. It often isn't reported until men are over the age of fifty.

Peyronie's disease is felt to be a wound healing disorder that occurs in those genetically susceptible men who have some form of injury to the penis. When it first starts, it often causes pain. This pain generally occurs during the inflammatory phase of the disease, which takes place during the first twelve to eighteen months of the disease. The exact etiology of this disease is unknown. The present theory believes that a man sustains repetitive minor trauma to the connective tissue layer. During the repair process, abnormal healing occurs. The disease is seen more commonly in diabetics, in men with hyperlipidemia (high cholesterol and/or triglycerides), smokers, males with Dupuytren's contracture (a genetic disease where the fingers of the hand develop contracture), and obesity.

The treatment for years has been topical vitamin E. Unfortunately, this treatment has not been shown to be that effective. It has continued because there appears to be little harm when using this topical treatment. Surgical correction, which does not always have a high success rate, can be considered in those instances where topical vitamin E has not helped and the penile deformity prevents a man from having an erection or having sexual penetration.

Ejaculatory Dysfunctions

You may have the equipment ready to fire your package, but how you release it can be flawed. There are two types of ejaculatory dysfunctions: retrograde ejaculation and premature ejaculation. Retrograde dysfunction is generally associated with a structural cause and premature ejaculation is usually due to an emotional cause.

Retrograde Ejaculation

Retrograde ejaculation occurs when the semen, instead of moving forward through the urethra to the end of the penis, moves backward into the bladder. Although you still reach sexual climax, you may ejaculate very little or no semen. This is sometimes called a dry orgasm. Your urine is often cloudy after an organism due to the semen in the urine. With lack of semen coming out forward at the time of an orgasm, it is one of the causes of male infertility. Retrograde ejaculation occurs when the bladder sphincter muscle does not close during ejaculation. This is often due to a nerve injury that can occur from prostate surgery, pelvic radiation, multiple sclerosis, spinal cord injury, or diabetes. If the nerve injury is severe, retrograde ejaculation may not be reversible and drugs often don't help. There are certain medications that can also cause retrograde ejaculation. The more common ones are certain blood pressure medications, drugs to treat mood disorders and alpha blockers, There are some medication that can used to try to treat retrograde ejaculation. They are Chlorpheniramine and brompheniramine (antihistaimines), imipramine (an antidepressant), and ephedrine or pseudoephedrine (decongestants).

Premature Ejaculation

If you have an ejaculation within one minute of attempting intercourse, it's considered premature ejaculation. Thirty percent of men with erectile dysfunction have premature ejaculation. It is often caused by performance anxiety, and it is commonly seen with anxious new explorers of sexual intimacy. To be classified as having premature ejaculation, a man must have all three of the following:

- A brief ejaculatory latency
- Loss of control of ejaculation
- A psychological distress because of this problem

The etiology of premature ejaculation can be divided into two main groups. The first group may have partners who has some type of sex-related problem, themselves. One such problem is a sexual pain syndrome, in which they may have pain during sex. The second group is the young anxious explorer of sex. He becomes so nervous at the time of his sexual encounter, he has premature ejaculation. I feel this happens more often than not. We would hear more about this, but young men are too embarrassed to admit that this happened to them. There is a simple technique that can help this: When you become excited and your glans penis (the head of the penis) becomes engorged and you feel close to ejaculating, you can grab under the glans penis and squeeze the penis. Often this breaks the crescendo towards ejaculating and slows down the process. If this does not work, you can discuss taking a trial of an SSRI medication with your doctor. These are the antidepressants that are in the Prozac family. Remember, these are the medications that have been shown to decrease libido and cause erectile dysfunction. When given in low doses, however, they have been shown to slow down the time before a person has an orgasm and therefore prevent premature ejaculation.

Infertility

Infertility is defined as the inability to achieve conception despite one year of frequent unprotected intercourse. Infertility is an aspect of sexuality that isn't discussed as often in men as it is in women. More often than not, if a couple is having problems trying to conceive, the finger is usually pointed at the woman. The reality is that about 20 percent of infertility problems are due to male infertility alone, and about 40 percent are due to a combination of problems with the man and the woman.

Causes of Male Infertility

More than 90 percent of male infertility cases are due to low sperm counts, poor sperm quality, or both. The remaining causes of male infertility can be due to a range of different conditions. These include anatomical problems, hormonal imbalances, and genetic defects.

Risk factors for male infertility include:

- Varicoceles—the enlarged spermatic veins in the spermatic cord that connects to the testicle. Guys who have varicoceles often refer to this as their "bag of worms." They are seen in 10 to 15 percent of normal men and in a higher percentage of infertile men. The warmth of the varicocele can affect the temperature around the sperm. This higher temperature may injure the developing sperm. This can be surgically corrected.

- Aging can reduce sperm counts and motility, which may decrease the genetic quality of the sperm.

- Sexually transmitted diseases can cause scarring in the male reproductive system or impair sperm function, which can cause infertility.

- Other causes of infertility are lifestyle factors, such as smoking and substance abuse. Also long-term or intensive exposure to certain types of chemicals, toxins, or medications can also cause problems procreating.

- Another more recent concern has been laptops. A few studies have revealed that usage of laptops has increased scrotal temperature like hot tubs, saunas, and jockey shorts. In theory at least, prolonged usage of laptops may contribute to infertility.

- Retrograde Ejaculation (discussed previously)

Diagnosing the Cause of Infertility

An evaluation begins with a complete medical exam. The history portion of the exam is extremely important. Has the man fathered children previously? If he has, then all systems had to be working in the past. If this is the case, what besides getting older (which, in itself, can be a potential cause of infertility) changed or occurred since then? Other important historical questions to examine are any past or present disease states. Diseases that affect a person's hormones can affect his fertility. What kinds of medications have been taken? This applies to medications in the past and present. Have there been any surgical procedures? This would include surgery to correct undescended testicles and obviously testicular removal. Some therapies, such as chemotherapy and radiation, can have long-lasting effects on a man's fertility.

The bottom line is to be sure to tell the doctor everything about your past medical history. Besides the normal physical exam, there needs to be a close inspection of the scrotum to see if there are signs of enlarged varicose veins. The following tests should be performed:

1. Semen analysis to evaluate the quantity and quality of sperm

2. Blood tests to evaluate hormone levels, including thyroid studies, TSH, T4, blood sugars, testosterone levels, and possibly prolactin levels if there is suspicion of a pituitary problem

3. Imaging tests if there is suspicion of structural problems

4. Genetic testing to identify sperm DNA fragmentation, chromosomal defects, or genetic diseases

Finally, there is also some suggestion that having high oxidative stress may damage sperm cells and may be an underlying cause in cases of unexplained infertility. Taking foods that have a high antioxidant effect, like all those colorful berries, could hopefully correct this.

Hypogonadism (Low Testosterone Production)

You can't turn on the TV these days without seeing a commercial discussing "Low T." The low T of course is low testosterone. When you watch those commercials, they give the impression that almost all men have low T. In reality it is more common than many of us in health care realized. I personally didn't believe that it was that common until I started reading the studies. As stated previously, a man's testosterone level starts to decrease after the age of thirty. The amount of decline is quite variable.

Some of the possible symptoms associated with low testosterone include:

- Decreased sexual drive

- Decreased spontaneous erections

- Loss of body hair

- Small testes

- Low sperm counts

- Low muscle mass

- Hot flashes*

- Loss of height, low bone density, and an increased fracture risk†

- Increased body fat‡

- Low energy

- Increased sadness/decreased joy

- Decreased strength

- Poor concentration and memory

- Disturbed sleep

- Decreased physical and work performance

---

* You may think only women experience this, but men with low testosterone can also have hot flashes. If low testosterone is due to a primary inability of the testicles to make enough testosterone, the brain senses the low level of testosterone. The brain will produce LH (luteinizing hormone) from the pituitary gland to stimulate testosterone production from the testicles. This is the same hormone that is produced by women to try to get their ovaries to make more estrogen during menopause. It is the LH that causes vasodilation and hot flashes.

† Testosterone is involved in the build up of bone in the body. Low testosterone impedes healthy bone formation.

‡ This occurs because a man who has low testosterone will have low muscle mass. With low muscle mass, the body has a tendency to have a lower metabolic rate and therefore a much higher likelihood of building up fat.

Occasionally, I am asked to perform a bone density and body composition scan on a guest at Canyon Ranch. Guests at Canyon Ranch can decide on their own if they want to obtain a body composition study (which looks at the percent of body fat and the amount of lean body muscle mass) and/or a bone density without first seeing a doctor. I was scheduled to obtain a bone density and body composition with the use of a dexa body scanner on a guest named Mitch. When I walked into the imaging room, I saw this 36-year-old young man who appeared overweight with an obvious paunch for a waistline. This is not unusual for many of my patients who visit Canyon Ranch. They often arrive because they are out of control with their health and may be overweight. They will come to Canyon Ranch to learn how to make changes in their lives both physically and emotionally. It appeared obvious to me that Mitch was another "typical" Canyon Ranch guest, who was here to get some baseline studies before embarking on a new healthy lifestyle.

I unfortunately put my foot in my mouth. I had assumed, after looking at Mitch, that he had not been taking care of himself. I felt there was no way with the shape of his body that he could be exercising on a regular basis. Whenever I have the chance to get someone to exercise, I will do it. After I made my preliminary introductions, I asked him if he was going to see one of our exercise experts to start an exercise program. As soon the words came out of my mouth, it was obvious that I had said something wrong. He appeared angry and immediately relayed to me that he was running on a regular basis. In fact, he had run six marathons in the previous three years! Boy did I fell like an idiot and apologized for assuming he wasn't exercising.

I proceeded with the bone density and body composition testing. The body composition revealed that he had 38 percent body fat, which certainly did not correlate with his running story. The real shock was his bone density. Before I came to Canyon Ranch, I felt only postmenopausal women should obtain a bone density study. I never thought it would be important for men to obtain one, because it's not considered a routine standard of care. In Mitch's case it was a huge eye-opener. Mitch himself had scheduled the bone density. When I performed the scan, I found out he had early signs of osteoporosis at the age of 36. So, here was this overweight marathoner who had signs of bone loss. What was going on? I explained to Mitch that this did not add up. I asked him if I could run some blood tests, and he willingly agreed to proceed.

What I found out was that he had a very low testosterone level, due to a premature testicular production failure. We started him on a topical testosterone, and in six months he had lost twelve pounds. He was shocked that it wasn't more, because his waist size decreased three inches and he looked great. It made obvious sense to me. With his higher level of testosterone, he was able to build up a significant amount of muscle mass. This larger muscle mass increased his metabolic rate, which in turn helped him burn more calories and lose fat. It is important to remember that muscle weighs more than fat. So even though he was losing fat from being able to build more muscle mass, he didn't lose as much total weight as he thought he would. Two years later his bone density was rechecked, and it was increasing in density and his body fat was 25 percent. As we can see with Mitch, testosterone is important for both muscle and bone growth.

Another more typical patient was Frank. He was 52 years of age and had been married for 20 years. He and his wife had attended my lecture on men's health. After the lecture, with a lot of encouragement from his wife, he decided to make an appointment to come in and see me. He stated that he had a two-year history of generalized fatigue and recently found out he was a borderline diabetic. His weight had gradually increased over the previous five years and now he was 30 pounds overweight. He had many more emotional down days than up days. His interest in sex had diminished, and he was having more episodes of not being able to obtain an erection.

On exam he was overweight; his waist size was 44 inches. No other significant abnormalities were noted. I obtained a body composition on him and found out he was 39 percent body fat and his lean body mass (muscle mass) was low. His blood work showed a low testosterone that was well below the reference range, and his HbA1C (this blood test measures blood sugar control over the previous three months) was elevated, which meant poor sugar control. In cases like this it is the classic "chicken or the egg" story. Did his elevated blood sugars affect his production of testosterone, or did his low testosterone elevate his blood sugar? Either way, his low testosterone had decreased his muscle mass. This in turn lowered his ability to burn calories.

After doing a thorough history and physical exam, including a cardiac workup, I decided to start him on a low dose topical testosterone, have him see a nutritionist, and start him on an exercise program. In four months he had dropped 25 pounds, his waist size decreased to 39 inches, and he had more energy than he had felt in years. His blood sugars improved and his interest in sex increased significantly. Even more important, his ability to obtain an erection had improved dramatically.

I would like to discuss the potential risk of cardiovascular disease when using testosterone to treat hypogonadism (low production of testosterone). In January 2014 there was a study published that revealed an increased risk of heart attacks and strokes for men over the age of 65 who took testosterone compared to those men who did not. As far as using testosterone in men under the age of 65, there was an increased risk of heart attacks or strokes if they had preexisting cardiovascular disease.[15]

Five months after that study was published (July of 2014) another article published in the *Annals of Pharmacotherapy* showed that older men who used testosterone had no increased risk of a heart attack.[16]

Finally, the most recent article that was published in JAMA at the time of the editing of this book showed that older men who were over the age of 60 (the average age was 67.6 years) who had low or low-normal testosterone and that were treated for three years with testosterone, showed no increased risk of developing cardiovascular disease.[17] This is confusing not only to you but also to the physicians who are writing the prescriptions. Women and their doctors have been in this position for years, trying to determine the safety of using hormone replacement therapy for menopausal symptoms. They had to worry about the potential of causing cancer or heart disease with hormone replacement therapy.

The decision on whether or not to treat a low testosterone level needs to be made between the doctor and the patient. Every case is different. If the individual is a young man with low testosterone, a poor sex drive, a decreased ability to obtain an erection, who has fatigue and mild depression, who is overweight and prediabetic, and has no heart disease, I would certainly support the usage of testosterone therapy. For men over the age of 60 with low testosterone there needs to be discussion with your doctor about all your symptoms which would include such things as decreased sex drive, weight gain, your sense of well-being and any past history of heart disease. These will all be taken into account in your decision with your doctor on whether or not you would be a candidate for testosterone therapy.

Performance-Enhancing Drugs

We have been looking at the positive effects that can occur when testosterone is given to men with low testosterone levels, but what about those individuals that are using it when they do not have a testosterone deficiency. This is a big part of what we call using performance enhancing drugs (PEDS). We all know about the professional athletes who have taken anabolic steroids to enhance their performance on the field. They are often tested and, if caught, can be banned or placed on probation from their chosen sport.

We need to be aware as parents that it isn't always the professional athletes that may be using these PEDS. It can be the high school athletes that are potentially ruining their lives from the use of these drugs There is so much pressure on winning and obtaining college scholarships, which are worth thousands of dollars that many teens are resorting to using PEDs. In one study they asked teenage boy athletes in Georgia if they were using some form of PEDs. Six percent admitted to using them.[18] This is a huge number, considering these drugs are illegal and the study was based on self-reporting. These performance-enhancing steroids can have severe and potentially long-lasting effects on health. Some of these side effects are reversible, while others are not. In growing adolescents one of the major risks of using anabolic steroid precursors is injury to the growth plates. Other side effects include shrunken testicles and breast growth in boys (gynecomastia). Boys may also experience acne and other health issues, such as: joint pain, tendon rupture, increased risk for forming blood clots, behavioral changes, liver dysfunction, and elevated blood pressures. Being aware as parents of teen boys using PEDS, and asking questions about their potential use with your sons and their coaches is the first step in addressing this problem.

A lot of ground is covered in the material presented in this chapter, but for a good reason. As discussed previously, men have a tendency to ignore their health, especially their sexual health. Because of this many men have had a large void in understanding this area. In fact many men have thought it was a sign of weakness to even discuss problems with their sexual health. Hopefully after reading this chapter the reader will now have greater insights and appreciation into their own sexual health.

10

Heart Health

We can't live without it.

H eart disease is the number one killer of men. (And for females reading this book, please note that heart disease, not breast cancer, is also the number one cause of death of women.)[19]

The heart disease that I will discuss in this chapter is coronary artery disease, which causes heart attacks. It is important to note that there are other types of heart disease, such as cardiomyopathy, which is a disease of the heart muscle itself. There is also valvular heart disease, in which the heart valves can be affected by a birth defect, infection, or the post infectious disease state called rheumatic fever.

A large percentage of what I do at Canyon Ranch is preventative medicine. This form of medicine has a simple premise: Determine the risk factors for a particular disease, and then try to eliminate those risk factors. Focusing on these risk factors often means cleaning up poor lifestyle habits. For some reason many men resist doing this. The "chore" of improved lifestyles appears difficult until they finally make the commitment to implement these changes. As I tell my patients, the lifestyle changes must become a "way of life." It's not a daily job but simply the path we follow each and every day of our lives.

When I examine the risk factors for heart disease, I look at which ones are modifiable and which ones are non-modifiable. The non-modifiable risk factors are those which a person has no control over and cannot change. (There is some argument about whether or not we have the potential of turning on and off genes, which is further explained in the chapter on epigenetics.) So, if you have a non-modifiable risk factor, meaning you can't do anything about it, why worry about it? The reason we need to know about the non-modifiable risk factors is that if someone has them then he needs to be more vigilant in addressing those risk factors he *can* control.

Non-Modifiable Risk Factors

Non-modifiable risk factors include family history, gender, age, and ethnic origin. When we speak of family history with heart disease, it can be rather vague. For example, would a third cousin who had heart disease count? The answer is no. The formal criteria states that there is an increased risk of having a heart attack if you have a family history of a first-degree blood relative (parent, sibling, or offspring) who has had heart attack or a stroke before the age of 55 if the person is a male relative, or before the age of 65 if the relative is a female. If there are more peripheral family members with heart disease or strokes, like an uncle, I don't ignore it, but consider it more of a relative increased risk than an absolute increased risk.

The next non-modifiable risk factor for having a heart attack is being a male. Men have a higher risk of heart disease than women. The older we are, the higher the probability there is of having heart risk. Finally, a person's ethnic origin is a non-modifiable risk factor for heart disease. Below are the average ages of death due to heart disease based on ethnic origin:[20]

- 65.3 years for Pacific Islanders
- 70.7 years for Native American Indians

- 71.3 years for African Americans
- 73.4 years for Hispanics
- 77.6 years for Asians
- 79.8 years for Caucasians

Modifiable Risk Factors

Modifiable risk factors are those factors that are known to increase the potential for having a heart attack. The big difference between this and the non-modifiable is that you can do something about these risk factors. A person can make changes in their lifestyles or simply stop certain unhealthy habits to decrease the risk for heart disease.

Smoking

The first and most obvious modifiable risk factor for heart disease is smoking.[21] I continue to be shocked at the number of men who still smoke. There has been so much in the media about the hazards of smoking that it is mind-boggling to me that anyone still does it. If you do smoke, QUIT!! There are too many tools out there to help you quit smoking, so please take advantage of them. Some of these tools include medication, hypnosis, and acupuncture. I am particularly biased towards acupuncture because I have been trained and certified in medical acupuncture. I have used acupuncture on my patients to quit smoking for more than fifteen years. I do not want to imply that acupuncture is the only way or the best way to quit smoking. Whichever treatment works for you, is the best way.

I became acquainted with a gentleman, Joe, who came to my office shortly after I started practicing acupuncture. His wife had sent him to see me to be treated with acupuncture to quit smoking. He admitted to me that he thought acupuncture was one of the stupidest things he had ever heard of. On a medical legal basis, I expressed to him that I thought it would be unwise for me to proceed with the acupuncture. To do an elective treatment on a person who had significant reservations about that treatment in the first place would be setting me up for disaster. If anything at all went wrong, I would certainly be blamed for it. I told him I would not charge him for the visit and he could go on his merry way back to his cigarettes.

He looked at me in absolute terror and said that if I did not proceed with this acupuncture treatment, his wife would kill him! He begged me to do it. I finally relented and proceeded with the treatment for smoking cessation. I told him to return in one week for a follow-up visit. When I said this, I was convinced this was the last time I was going to see this gentleman.

To my amazement Joe returned a week later for another session. I told him I was surprised to see him again. He told me that he really couldn't understand it. Two days after I had treated him, he had to take a load of goods for his work 100 miles away. Every week he made this trek with his coworker, Bill. Between the two of them, they usually smoked at least two packs of cigarettes. He said on the way up to the drop-off site, he realized he didn't want to smoke. Every time his friend would offer him a cigarette, he turned it down. His friend kept asking him if he was okay. For the rest of the week, he didn't smoke a cigarette. Because of this incredible result, he—not his wife—made the decision to return for a second treatment. This treatment success by itself showed me how effective acupuncture could be for smoking cessation.

High Blood Pressure

Another modifiable risk factor for coronary heart disease is high blood pressure.[22] The definition of high blood pressure has changed over the years. Most recently, the Joint National Commission on Hypertension (JNC8)[23] stated in 2013 that below age 60, high blood pressure is defined as pressures 140/90 and higher. At the age of 60 or older, high blood pressure is defined as pressures 150/90 and higher, unless the person has chronic kidney disease or diabetes. In that case the diagnosis of high blood pressure remains at 140/90 and higher. At the time of publishing this book, new studies are suggesting our blood pressure should be less than 120/80. Uncontrolled high blood pressure can injure blood vessel walls and start the cascade of events that can lead to plaque (blockages in the arteries) formation. This can cause heart attacks and strokes. There are other disease states that can occur with uncontrolled high blood pressure; it is a leading cause of heart failure and kidney failure.

Testing your blood pressure is simple. You don't have to go to your doctor's office to have it checked. The best way to monitor your blood pressure is to do it yourself with one of the many self-monitoring blood pressure machines that are available at your local pharmacy or through the Internet. Some of the new blood-pressure monitors attach right to your smartphone. I am often asked when the best time is to check your blood pressure. The answer is that it needs to be checked throughout the day. The blood pressure that a physician uses to determine if you have hypertension (abnormally elevated blood pressures) is the average of your daily blood pressure readings. Beware of this if you have a slight OCD (obsessive compulsive disorder). I have seen some people become so obsessed with checking their blood pressure that their anxiety causes them to have an artificially elevated blood pressure.

Not everyone who has high blood pressure needs medication. Often lifestyle changes can treat high blood pressure. For example, if you are overweight, lose the weight. Being overweight can often lead to high blood pressure—especially if you have excessive belly fat. Belly fat acts like an endocrine organ. It can produce a chemical called angiotensin. For years we have known angiotensin was produced in the kidneys to regulate your blood pressure. Its job is to elevate your blood pressure whenever your blood pressure drops, such as when you become dehydrated or have some type of blood loss. Angiotensin is a vasoconstrictor, which causes the arterial walls to contract, elevating your blood pressure.

It has now been discovered that belly fat has the capability of producing angiotensin. Angiotensin produced from belly fat doesn't respond to the body's fluid status or blood pressure—it just keeps making more angiotensin. With the overproduction of angiotensin from an individual's belly fat, blood pressure will rise. One of the commonly used medications for high blood pressure is ACE inhibitors, such as lisenopril and accupril, which block the production of angiotensin in the body. They are an effective medication with few side effects. If you have high blood pressure and belly fat, a better strategy than using medication to lower the blood pressure is simply to decrease the belly fat. Patients often ask me how they can get off their blood pressure medications. This is a true example of cause and effect. The cause for the high blood pressure is often the overproduction of angiotensin from belly fat, and the simple answer is weight loss, not a pill.

Inflammation

Elevated levels of inflammation in the body is another modifiable risk factor that can cause heart disease.[24] This is a hard concept to understand, because excessive inflammation can come from many sources. The sources may be a chronic infection such as gingivitis, an acute infection like a cold virus, an autoimmune disease like rheumatoid arthritis, or a heightened immune system. If this elevated level of inflammation is not transient, like during a cold virus, but is persistent, there is an increased risk for cardiovascular disease. For this reason it is important to treat persistent inflammation in the body. If you have bad teeth or gums, see a dentist (better yet, obtain regular dental checkups so you don't develop the inflammation in the first place). If your rheumatoid arthritis is not in remission, treat it aggressively with your rheumatologist to get it under better control.

Another major source for excessive inflammation in the body is belly fat. It is a warehouse of unwanted chemicals in the body. We

Strength Training with Bands

You may not always have easy access to weights. A very simple and effective way to weight train without weights is to use elastic bands. Exercise elastic band sets can be purchased from most athletic supply stores or through Amazon. Shown here are some strength training exercises using the elastic bands. All three of these exercises are to be performed with both feet standing on the middle portion of the elastic band.

Exercise 1: Squat to Stand

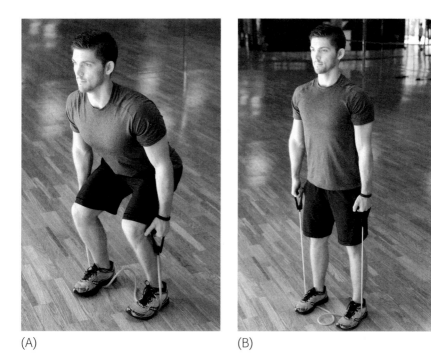

(A) (B)

From a squatting position grasp the ends of an elastic band, and then stand to return to a vertical position. Repeat this 10 times.

Exercise 2: Squat Pull to Squat Relax

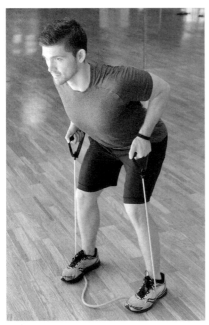

(A)

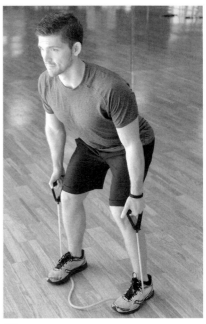

(B)

In a squatting position and with arms extended, pull the bands up by flexing the arms but remaining in the squatting position. Repeat this 10 times.

Exercise 3: Standing Arm Flex and Arm Extended

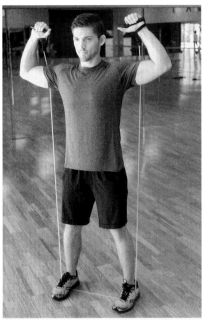

(A)

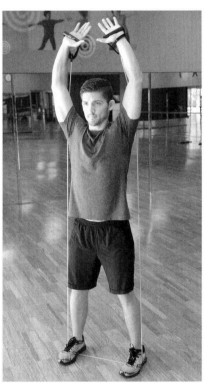

(B)

Starting from the standing position and the arms flexed above the head, pull the bands upward and extend the arms. Repeat this 10 times.

Balance Exercises

In addition to strength training, there are several exercises that can be practiced to help improve a person's balance. Here are a few of these exercises that can be done without equipment.

Exercise 1: Standing on one leg with arms and hands in anatomical position

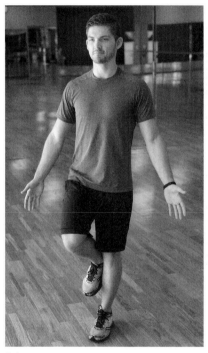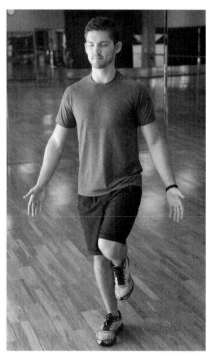

(A)   (B) Eyes closed

Stand on one leg. Flex opposite leg and extend arms on both sides. Stand on each leg for a minimum of 30 seconds. To make it more challenging, close your eyes during the exercise.

Exercise 2: Reaching for object on one foot: standing prior to reaching, and reaching for object

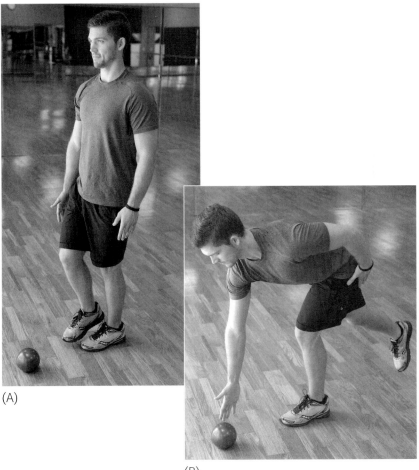

(A)

(B)

From an upright position and standing on one leg, lean forward and touch an object with the hand of the opposite side as the supporting leg. Repeat this 10 times. Then perform the same thing on the opposite side 10 times.

Exercise 3: Leaning to one side while standing on one leg

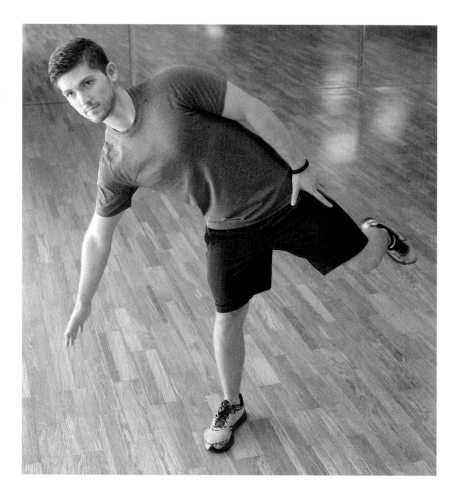

For a more difficult balancing exercise, stand on one leg and lean sideways (on the same side as the supporting leg) for 30 seconds; then do the same thing on the opposite side.

Exercise 4: Advanced balance exercise with extended arm and extended opposite leg

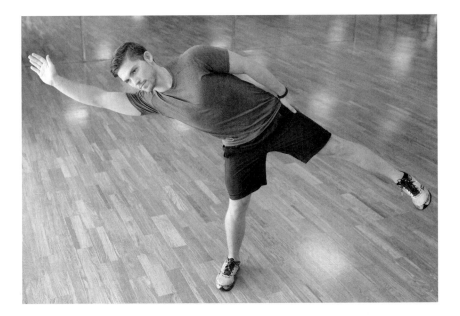

For a more advanced balancing exercise, stand on one leg, extend the arm on the same side as the standing leg, and then with the free leg straighten it out. Do this for 30 seconds. Then repeat this exercise on the opposite side.

Simple Morning Stretching Exercises

There are several advantages to stretching: it can decrease injuries, and it can help relieve musculoskeletal pain that is seen with arthritis, fibromyalgia, and chronic back pain. It is also helpful in improving balance, flexibility, and coordination. It is important to stretch prior to exercising and immediately after exercising when your muscles are heated up.

The following are simple stretching exercises that can be done at any age and are a good way to begin your day.

Exercise 1: Arms extended overhead in standing position

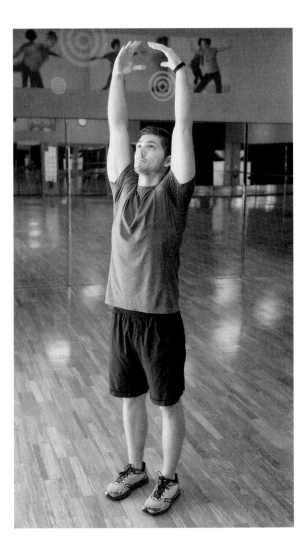

Stretch arms overhead for 30 seconds.

Exercise 2: Arms extended behind the person

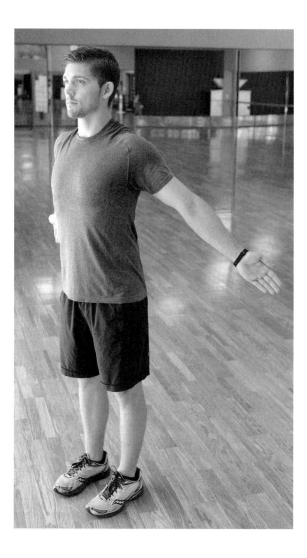

In a standing position extend the arms behind you for 30 seconds.

Exercise 3: On the floor with legs extended and grasping the ankles

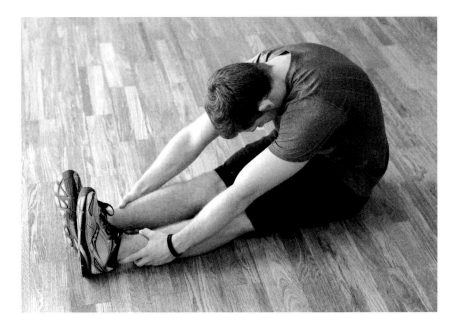

In the sitting position with the legs extended, gasp behind the legs with your hands as far down the legs as you can and hold it for 30 seconds.

Progressive Muscular Relaxation

Progressive Muscular Relaxation is an exercise to help with stress. The technique is performed first by lying down on your back in a relaxed state. Next, contract the upper body muscles for 30 seconds. Then relax those muscles for 30 seconds. Then contract the mid-region muscles for 30 seconds followed by relaxing those muscles for 30 seconds. Finally contract the muscles of the lower body for 30 seconds. Then relax them for 30 seconds. You can repeat this process more than once.

Exercise 1: Relaxed and supine

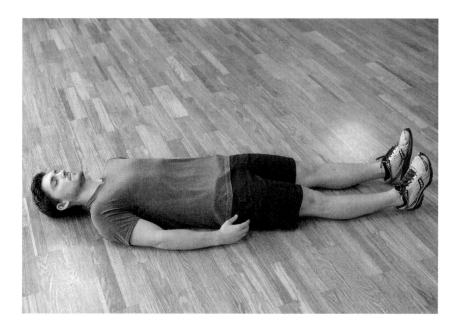

Relaxed position lying down.

Exercise 2: Upper body and face contraction

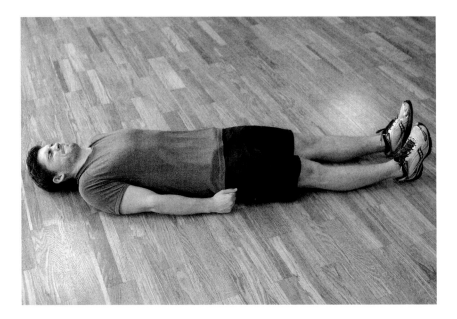

Contracting the upper body.

Exercise 3: Mid-body contraction

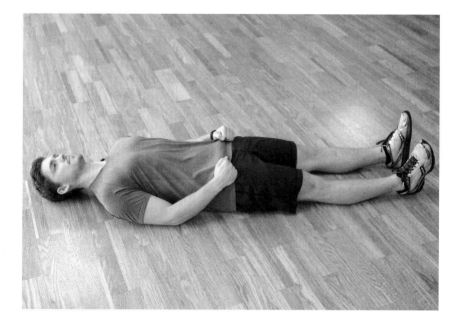

Contracting the mid-body.

Exercise 4: Lower body contraction

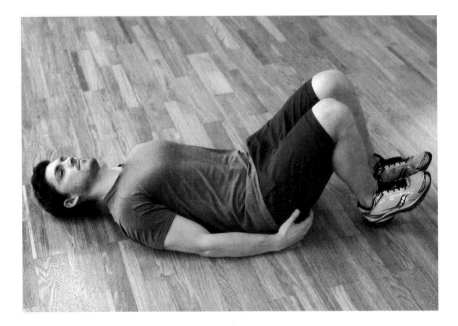

Contracting the lower body.

already learned that belly fat is capable of producing a chemical called angiotensin, which can cause elevated blood pressure. It also has the potential of producing excessive amounts of chemicals in the body called cytokines. Two notable cytokines are interleukin-6 and tissue necrosis factor-alpha. Cytokines are involved in many inflammatory reactions in the body. Having inflammation in the body is not always a bad thing—it can be used to rid our body of foreign objects, such as bad bacteria. If you don't have an infection, however, these little knights in shining armor can turn into little Darth Vaders. Inflammation has the potential of injuring good tissue in our bodies, notably the walls of our arteries. This injury can potentially lead to a progression of events causing plaque formation.

The good news is that there is a blood test to measure the amount of inflammation in the body; it is called the C-reactive protein. Many of the lab's reference ranges state that the goal is to be under 3 nanograms/milliliter. Our goal at Canyon Ranch is to be fewer than 0.7 nanograms/milliliter. Studies have shown that higher levels (greater than 0.7 nanograms/milliliter) of C-reactive protein increase the risk for cardiovascular disease. A word of caution: This test is very sensitive and a simple cold virus can cause the C-reactive protein to be temporarily elevated. This is a normal response and as long as the C-reactive protein drops back down to its pre-viral state, there will be no increased cardiovascular risks.

There are lifestyle changes that can lower your CRP. Regular moderate to high-intensity exercise can lower your CRP with or without weight loss.[25] Also what you eat may alter your CPR. Changing your diet to more polyunsaturated fat diet with less saturated fats can lower your CRP. It has the best effect of lowering CRP if the polyunsaturated fats has a lower content of omega-6s (examples of omega-6s are: sunflower, safflower, soy, sesame, and corn oils).[26]

Cholesterol

Another major risk factor for developing heart disease is elevated levels of cholesterol.[27] By now most of you have learned that there is "good" and "bad" cholesterol. I would like to shine a more comprehensive light on this. There are two major forms of fat in the body: cholesterol and triglycerides. Cholesterol is an essential structural component of animal cell membranes, and it serves as a precursor for the biosynthesis of steroid hormones, bile acids, and vitamin D. Triglycerides are the chief storage form of fat in the body. Because fats are insoluble in water, they are also insoluble in blood. In order to transport these fats through the blood stream, they have to be made water-soluble. This is accomplished by using fat carriers called lipoproteins, which are a combination of a fat and protein molecule. The protein surrounds the fat and makes it soluble in water. There are several types of lipoproteins, including:

- **HDL** (high density lipoprotein): carries cholesterol

- **LDL** (low density lipoprotein): carries cholesterol

- **VLDL** (very low density lipoprotein): carries triglycerides

- **IDL** (intermediate density lipoprotein): carries triglycerides and cholesterol

The "good" cholesterol is HDL, which transports cholesterol away from the arteries and toward the liver to rid the body of excess cholesterol. The "bad" cholesterol is LDL, which transports cholesterol toward the arteries. What has been considered healthy and a lower risk of heart disease is having a high level of HDL and a low level of LDL. This is true, but unfortunately it can miss a certain percentage of high-risk patients.

As you can see, VLDL carries triglycerides and IDL carries both cholesterol and triglycerides. If you only look at LDL and HDL, you will miss a certain percentage of high-risk patients for heart disease. The good news is that one protein, apolipoprotein B, is the protein found in LDL, IDL, and VLDL. These transport cholesterol and triglycerides toward the arteries. Only one protein, apolipoprotein A1, is in the carrier of the "good" cholesterol, HDL. If you check an apolipoprotein B level and apolipoprotein A1 level, these two proteins can give you a much better overall picture of your healthy or nonhealthy cholesterol status. This was proven in the AMORIS study, which looked at 175,000 individuals in Sweden and found out that apolipoprotein B blood levels were a better predictor of atherosclerotic (hardening of the arteries) cardiovascular disease than LDL.[28] In addition, it was noted that the ratio of apolipoprotein B to apolipoprotein A1 was also an excellent predictor of atherosclerotic heart disease. For this reason, I often obtain an apolipoprotein A1 and B level during my routine cholesterol studies.

For many years, people have been prescribed a diet low in saturated fats to lower cholesterol.[29] Saturated fats are solid fats like butter, lard, and meat fats. The word saturated means the fat is saturated with hydrogen atoms, which makes it solid (unsaturated fats contain less hydrogen atoms and are in a liquid state like soybean oil, olive oil, and corn oil). Saturated fats have been shown to increase LDL cholesterol (and to a minor degree also increase HDL cholesterol). Because high LDL cholesterol levels have been associated with increased heart disease risk,[30] the national guidelines in the U.S. tried to simplify things by reducing all fats despite little or no evidence that it actually prevented heart disease. This was the dawn of all the low-fat diets. The bottom line is that all fats are not alike. Polyunsaturated fatty acids, for example, are a fat but they can actually lower a person's LDL cholesterol and raise their HDL cholesterol.

The other problem that can occur when we attempt to eliminate all fats is that we replace them with sugars. These concentrated carbs can cause rapid elevations of blood sugar. The body responds to this by producing a spike in insulin. High levels of insulin in turn increase the storage of fat and at the same time lower blood sugar levels quickly. With rapid lowering of the blood sugar, there is increased hunger and resultant increased food consumption. That of course often leads to weight gain.

The last piece on fats, which is rapidly becoming a non-issue, is trans fats. They are now being eliminated from our diets, as the result of the work accomplished by the FDA, whose comment on trans fats is that they are generally considered to be unsafe.[31] Trans fats are formed by taking a liquid polyunsaturated fat (for example, corn oil) and turning it into a solid by heating the oil and adding hydrogen atoms to it. Trans fats are considered to be an increased risk for heart disease because of their effect on the lipoproteins LDL and HDL. Trans fats have the tendency to increase a person's LDL and decrease their HDL.

Often there is a strong family history of heart disease without obvious risk factors (smoking, elevated cholesterol, high blood pressure, and so on). If this is the case, I will order a test that breaks down cholesterol particles more deeply than the LDL and HDL. This test looks at the different sizes of LDL and HDL cholesterol. In other words, not all cholesterol is alike. Cholesterol particle sizes aren't routinely checked during a cholesterol blood draw, so you may need to ask your doctor to run this test. Smaller cholesterol particles can be more damaging to the arterial walls and increase the risk of forming plaque.

One of those important small particles is called Lp(a) cholesterol, and it is highly associated with atherosclerosis and coronary artery disease.[32] This particular LDL cholesterol is like the neutron bomb of LDL particles. It is this tiny piercing LDL that loves to slam into the artery wall and cause damage, which sets up events leading to the hardening of your arteries. If your level is high, the treatment is somewhat controversial. Some cardiologists feel you should treat it with niacin, and other cardiologists feel you need to lower your overall LDL cholesterol to less than 70. Aspirin has also been shown to help lower it. The bottom line is that an elevated level of Lp(a) in itself is an increased cardiovascular risk factor.

Since I work at Canyon Ranch and my subspecialty is Integrative Medicine, I try to improve health by lifestyle changes before I prescribe medications. Because of this, I am often asked if I write prescriptions for statin medications (Lipitor, Crestor, Zocor, and so on). The answer is yes. Statins are not a perfect medication. I have seen many patients complain of muscle pains with these drugs (despite what a recent study said disputing this). Other potential side effects include liver inflammation and occasional elevated blood sugars. Despite the potential side effects associated with statins, one cannot ignore the evidence that they have decreased heart disease. With the barrage of TV advertising promoting the usage of statins, one would think that the effect of taking a statin would decrease your risk of having a heart attack by a huge percentage. The reality is it does decrease your risk but not by as much as they want you to believe.

I will prescribe a statin to a patient if:

- They have had a past history of a cardiovascular event (like a stroke or heart attack).

- They are diabetic (Even though statins have been shown to occasionally increase a person's blood sugar level, they have been shown to be particularly effective in lowering the risk of heart disease in diabetics.[33]

- They show signs of plaque formation (noted by imaging studies, such as carotid ultrasound or a CT heart scan) and are unable to get their cholesterol down to the therapeutic range (LDL < 70 mg/dl).

- They have high cholesterol levels and are unable to lower their cholesterol (generally the goal is an LDL of < 100 mg/dl) after at least a three-month trial of diet and exercise.

Statins, because they have been so successful in lowering cholesterol, have become a multibillion-dollar windfall for the pharmaceutical companies. This has resulted in a constant multimedia blitz to the public to promote them. This media blitz has caused people to think that cholesterol is now the only risk factor we need to consider in preventing heart disease. Please do not fall into this trap. A recent large study (approximately 95,000 participants) demonstrated that 50 percent of individuals who had a heart attack or stroke were found to have normal cholesterol levels.[34] This study alone reveals that cholesterol is not the only risk factor in heart disease. Please do not ignore the other cardiovascular risk factors.

Elevated Blood Sugars

Another risk factor for coronary heart disease is elevated blood sugars. Diabetes doubles the risk for cardiovascular disease in men. Even the pre-diabetic state, called the metabolic syndrome, has been shown to increase the risk for cardiovascular disease. This pre-diabetic state is defined as having three of the following five indicators:

- Abdominal obesity; a waist circumference in men ≥102 cm (40 in) and in women ≥88 cm (35 in)
- Serum triglycerides ≥150 mg/dL (1.7 mmol/L) or on drug treatment for elevated triglycerides
- Serum HDL cholesterol <40 mg/dL (1 mmol/L) in men and <50 mg/dL (1.3 mmol/L) in women
- Blood pressure ≥140/90 mmHg or on a drug treatment for elevated blood pressure

- Fasting plasma glucose ≥100 mg/dL (5.6 mmol/L). If you are greater than 125 mg/dl, you are already a diabetic.

Elevation of blood sugars can lead to changes in the lining of the blood vessel wall, called the endothelium, by lowering nitric oxide levels. Nitric oxide is one of the more important molecules synthesized by the endothelium. It causes vascular dilation, prevents blood clotting, and inhibits an inflammatory response in the wall of the vessel.

Diabetes is treatable, but even when glucose levels are under control, there is an increased risk of heart disease and stroke. This increased risk, particularly in type II diabetes, may be due to the fact that these individuals often have associated high blood pressure, obesity, and elevated lipids (cholesterol and triglycerides). Diabetics often have high LDL cholesterol, low HDL cholesterol, and high triglycerides. This pattern of lipid profile is often seen in patients with premature coronary heart disease.

Being Overweight or Obese

This has long been known to be a risk factor for cardiovascular disease. This increased risk is due to several mechanisms, which includes hypertension, inflammation, and insulin resistance. Weight loss is often the simple solution to this risk factor.

Physical Inactivity

- World Health Organization believes that more than 60 percent of the global population is not sufficiently active.

- Physical activity protects you by regulating your weight and improving insulin sensitivity and blood sugar control.

- Being active is beneficial for your blood pressure, blood lipid levels, blood clotting factors, and lowering inflammation.

- Studies show that doing more than 150 minutes per week of moderate physical activity will reduce your risk of coronary heart disease by about 30 percent.

Biology of Vascular Disease

In this chapter we have been looking at factors that increase the risk of forming atherosclerosis (plaque build-up in the arteries). How can we detect prior to an event (such as having a heart attack) if the process of atherosclerosis has already started? One way is imaging a person's arteries, which can be done in various ways. A CT scan of the heart can indicate the presence of plaque by detecting calcium deposition in the coronary arteries. The drawback of the CT scan is that it produces a significant amount of radiation. The other problem with a CT scan is that if you are less than sixty years of age, you may miss some plaque formation because calcium tends to deposit later in the evolution of plaque.

Another form of imaging that is helpful in determining plaque development is a carotid ultrasound. No, this is not looking directly at the coronary arteries, but disease in the carotid arteries is often highly correlated with what is occurring in the coronary arteries. It can pick up arterial wall changes much earlier than a CT heart scan, sometimes even with individuals in their twenties. It is important to have an experienced ultrasonographer to look for plaque formation and thickening of the arterial walls. Both of these are associated with atherosclerosis.

Imaging is a great help in determining if plaque has formed. However, there are certain biochemical blood markers that, when present in the body, may indicate that plaque is actively forming. These specialized blood tests can be obtained in commercial labs. One of those labs is Cleveland HeartLabs, which measures the following blood levels:

- **F2 Isoprostanes.** This is an excellent way of measuring oxidative stress in the body. High levels of oxidative stress are disruptive to cells and over time can increase the risk of chronic disease. It acts as a very strong vasoconstrictor and can increase the risk of developing blood clots.[35]

- The second important biomarker is **oxidized LDL.** This is formed when the protein of LDL cholesterol, apolipoprotein B, becomes oxidized. It has the potential of causing significant damage to the blood vessel wall. Scavenger white blood cells (called macrophages) swallow up oxidized LDL, forming what is called a foam cell in the blood vessel wall. This initiates an inflammatory response in the arterial wall. In healthy middle-aged men, high oxidized LDL is associated with a four times higher risk of developing coronary artery disease.[36] In addition, it has been found that individuals with elevated oxidized LDL are also at a much higher risk for developing the pre-diabetic state called metabolic syndrome that was discussed earlier.

- Another indicator of active vascular disease is **the presence of microscopic protein in the urine.** Generally, for this to take place, there needs to be damage to the small blood vessels in the kidney. If damage is occurring in the blood vessels to the kidney, there is then a high probability that injury has occurred in other blood vessels in the body.[37]

- There are two cardiac biomarkers that are highly associated with active disease; they are **Lp-PLA2**[38] and **Myeloperoxidase (MPO).**[39] Lp-PLA2 or lipoprotein-associated phospholipase-A2 is a vascular-specific inflammatory enzyme that helps form plaque. The Lp-PLA2 particle enters an artery wall bound to LDL cholesterol. It modifies oxidized LDL, causing it to increase inflammation. The old version of understanding atherosclerosis is that there is a slow build-up of cholesterol plaque in the artery walls. The more recent explanation that the condition is one of an inflamed section of your artery that swells like a volcano. If left unchecked it can enlarge and finally explode, sending particles downstream. These exploding particles can acutely clog up your artery and cause a heart attack or stroke. The other biomarker at this near explosive phase is myeloperoxidase (MPO). If you have an elevation of MPO, you are more than twice as likely to die of a heart attack compared to the rest of the population. MPO also oxidizes LDL and causes LDL to deposit in the arteries directly forming plaque. MPO in addition decreases a person's nitric oxide, which as we learned earlier, is involved in blood vessel dilation.

Heart disease is the number one cause of death in men. The good news is there are a lot of things a person can do to decrease their risk of developing heart disease. This can be done by minimizing or eliminating modifiable risk factors such as unhealthy habits, like smoking, and by addressing and correcting abnormal blood chemistries such as elevated cholesterol and increased CRP.

11

Prostate Cancer

The second leading cause of cancer death in men

There is a common belief among many men that prostate cancer is a natural progression of aging and if they live long enough they will all develop prostate cancer. Men also say that prostate cancer rarely kills anyone. This is a false perception because prostate cancer is the second leading cause of cancer death in men. Only lung cancer kills more men each year. Men have done a poor job of educating each other about this disease. Women, on the other hand, have been very successful in breast cancer awareness compared to prostate cancer awareness. They have accomplished this through such programs as the Susan B. Komen Breast Cancer runs and having pink ribbon campaigns. Interestingly, the lifetime risk of a women developing breast cancer is 13 percent and the lifetime risk of a man developing prostate cancer is 16 percent.

Risk Factors for Prostate Cancer

There are several risk factors for developing prostate cancer. The first is age. Sixty-three percent of prostate cancers occur in men over the age of sixty-five. Other risk factors are race, family history, obesity, and possibly diet. In the United States, African Americans have the highest incidence of prostate cancer. Asians and Native Americans have the lowest incidence.[40] With family history it is not only the obvious first-degree relative with prostate cancer (father or brother)[41] but also if you have a family history of the BRCA1[42] or BRCA2[43] gene mutation or a strong history of women with breast cancer.

Early Detection with PSA

Each year more and more men are being diagnosed with prostate cancer. It was originally feared that the actual incidence of the disease was increasing. That appears not to be the case. The increased numbers of prostate cancers are due to the widespread usage of the biomarker PSA (prostate surface antigen). This has resulted in the detection of prostate cancer in more men at much earlier stages.

The PSA is a protein produced by cells of the prostate gland. There are three things that can increase a man's PSA. The first and most common is simply an enlargement of the prostate. This is called benign prostatic hypertrophy (discussed earlier). The second is an infection of the prostate, which is called prostatitis (discussed previously). The third is prostate cancer. Since there are reasons other than prostate cancer that can cause the PSA to elevate, the PSA alone cannot be used to detect prostate cancer. A prostate biopsy is the only way to make a definitive diagnosis.

What is considered to be a "normal" PSA level? The standard answer is fewer than 4.0 nanograms/milliliter. It is important to know that this is not a hard and fast rule. This was seen in the Prostate Cancer Prevention Trial that was funded by the National Cancer Institute.[44] In this study 18,000 men ages 55 and older were followed over time. At the end of the study, they were given a prostate biopsy. Of the men diagnosed with prostate cancer, 21 percent had a PSA level between 2.6 and 3.9 ng/ml. On the other hand a PSA greater than 4.0 nanograms/milliliter does not mean you have prostate cancer. In a study that looked at PSAs greater than 4.0 nanograms/milliliter, only 25 percent of men who had a PSA level between 4.0 and 10.0 nanograms/milliliter had biopsy proven prostate cancer.[45] This meant that 75 percent of the remaining men did not have prostate cancer. So the absolute PSA number is not always the key to a diagnosis of prostate cancer. The trends in a man's PSA over time is often more significant in making a prostate cancer diagnosis than the absolute number. That is why it is important to obtain regular PSAs to note any sudden increase in PSA levels. (A recent study tried to dispute this, however most physicians feel trending is very helpful.)[46] If a man has been having yearly PSAs in the 1.0 range and then suddenly it jumps to 2.8, I will not ignore it, even though it is still well below 4.0. I would first recheck the blood level to see if it really is elevated, and then look into potential pathologic causes for that jump. These could include prostate infection as well as prostate cancer.

When should a man first obtain a PSA and how often should the test be performed? This is controversial. I feel men should obtain a PSA starting at the age of 50 and then have it checked yearly after that. If there is a family history of prostate cancer, or if they are African American, I will obtain PSAs at the age of 40. I have seen enough men who were diagnosed with prostate cancer in their forties to warrant having it done at this age. Is it the smartest medical expenditure? The answer is probably no—unless you were the one who was diagnosed with early prostate cancer.

I feel it is important to discuss the recommendations from the United States Preventative Services Task Force.* The U.S. Preventative Services Task Force has recommended that men not have a yearly

---

* Created in 1984, the U.S. Preventive Services Task Force (USPSTF or Task Force) is an independent group of national experts in prevention and evidence-based medicine that works to improve the health of all Americans by making evidence-based recommendations about clinical preventive services such as screenings, counseling services, or preventive medications.

PSA. They feel the test is less reliable as we age, especially in men over the age of 75. The increased size of the prostate produces more prostatic proteins that can gradually elevate a man's PSA. With this rise there is often an obligation to proceed with a biopsy, which can be painful and has the potential for complications. If the biopsy is positive then the man must determine his treatment options, which can lead to other additional complications. The U.S. Preventative Services Task Force feels that men should not have to endure this pain and stress. As much as I appreciate all the great work the U.S. Preventative Services Task Force has completed in this area to prevent unnecessary procedures, I still feel the final decision on when a person can and should obtain a PSA needs to be between the patient and his doctor, not the U.S. Preventative Services Task Force.

There has been a push by those who are both "fiscally responsible" and advocates in preventing unnecessary procedures to limit the use of PSAs, and in some cases consider eliminating PSAs altogether. They feel the yearly PSAs will lead to excessive medical costs and unwarranted procedures. The "fiscally responsible" in their zeal to eliminate yearly PSAs will often use the argument that if every man lives long enough, he will eventually develop prostate cancer. If you follow that argument, then you could use the same verbiage for heart disease. If every man lives long enough, he will develop heart disease. So why treat or try to prevent heart disease?

During my first years of practicing medicine (which started in 1982), I never made a diagnosis of early onset prostate cancer. When I did make a diagnosis of prostate cancer in a patient, it was always at an advanced stage. By that time there was little chance of a cure. The only treatments we had to offer were palliative. This usually meant pain relief and treatment for the complications associated with metastatic disease, such as bone fractures. In those days prior to the usage of the PSA as a diagnostic tool, the only way to make a diagnosis of prostate cancer was in one of three ways: by performing a rectal exam and feeling a rock hard prostate, if the patient's symptoms were associated with some type of urinary obstruction (difficulty starting urination, getting up multiple times at night to urinate, and so on) or if the patient presented with signs of metastatic spread, such as unrelenting lower back pain due to a spread of the cancer to the bones.

Nowadays, we think of obtaining a PSA as a diagnostic tool for early detection of prostate cancer. That was not the intended use of this biomarker. Its original use was to help oncologists or urologists determine if their therapy to treat an already diagnosed prostate cancer was effective. The physician would obtain a PSA prior to treatment and would then recheck a PSA after therapy for the cancer. If the patient's PSA dropped, that meant the cancer therapy had some effect on the cancer. In the mid-1990s, I wondered to myself if we could use the PSA not only as a tumor marker, in determining the efficacy of a cancer treatment, but also as a diagnostic tool for early prostate cancer detection. I remember talking to urologists at the time, and they thought it was a crazy idea. I decided to do it anyway.

I remember the day about twenty years ago when I obtained a PSA on Bob, who was a government worker in his early fifties. He took early retirement and was going to move to Colorado and spend his golden years enjoying the mountains with his wife. He came to my office for a complete physical before leaving town, so he could put one last medical bill on good old Uncle Sam. I decided to perform a PSA as part of his routine blood work. He had never had this test before. It was mildly elevated, and I told him that it was a little higher than what I wanted to see. I repeated the test and it remained above normal. I advised him to see a urologist. He reluctantly went, and the urologist asked him why he'd been referred. My patient relayed that it was because he had an abnormal PSA. At that time the urologist thought it was unnecessary to be seen just because Bob had a slightly elevated PSA, but he again repeated the test and it remained elevated. The urologist said he was "obligated" to proceed with a prostate biopsy, even though the rectal exam showed no prostatic abnormalities. The biopsy was not only positive for prostate cancer but also it was an extremely aggressive type. The urologist proceeded with a surgical excision of the prostate. Bob tolerated the procedure well and had no post-operative complications. Every year I still receive a Christmas card from Bob telling me he is still around, hiking in the mountains of Colorado.

Treating Prostate Cancer

Surgical treatment for prostate cancer does not cause the obvious physical changes to the body that a mastectomy does for women. However, the treatment has the potential of causing significant functional changes in the body, such as urinary incontinence and impotence. This can lead to obvious emotional distress. These quality of life issues are a large part in the decision-making process of how a man chooses to treat his prostate cancer.

When looking at a prostate cancer biopsy, a pathologist grades the aggressiveness of the tumor by giving it a Gleason score. This number will be between 1 and 10. The higher the number, the more aggressive the tumor. This number is important when discussing treatment options with your doctor.

Medicine is so rapidly changing in relation to cancer therapies that it is impossible to know if they will be modified or changed by the time this book is published. With that in mind, I'll address some of the current treatments now available. There are basically five different avenues in the treatment of prostate cancer:

- Active Surveillance
- Surgical Prostatectomy

- Radiation Therapy
- Androgen (Male Hormone) Deprivation Therapy
- Watchful Waiting

The decision on which course to take is between the patient, the doctor, and often the patient's intimate partner. The ultimate decision maker is the patient. He is the one who must live with the consequences of treatment or no treatment. There are many variables in making the decision on how to treat this disease. I am a firm believer in getting as much information as possible beforehand. The man's first decision is if he should have therapy in the first place and if it should be made before obtaining a PSA. As noted earlier, some people believe that after a certain age a PSA test should not be administered. Certainly, if you are a relatively healthy 82-year-old man, one may question the wisdom of obtaining a PSA. I still think it would be reasonable to obtain a PSA on that 82-year-old if he presented with a new-onset, debilitating lower back pain, without any known injury. If the PSA were high, then a diagnosis of metastatic prostate cancer would be high on the list of diagnostic possibilities. Knowing that prostate cancer was the most likely cause of the pain would make it easier to not necessarily cure the patient, but to at least offer him effective palliative care to improve his quality of life.

Active Surveillance

Let's look at the first therapy option. Active Surveillance is defined as the postponement of immediate therapy, with a curative-intent treatment instituted if there is evidence of disease progression. It may be considered in a small, well-differentiated prostate cancer that has a relatively low risk of progression. (This is different from "watchful waiting," which will be discussed later.) These men may be active sexually, and they do not want to have any therapy that has the possibility of disrupting their sexual activity by causing impotence or potentially causing bladder dysfunction, such as incontinence. But if there are signs of disease progression, then an aggressive treatment can still be instigated at the choice of the patient.

Radical Prostatectomy

With this option, there is hope for a cure. It is, as the word implies, radical. The focus is to remove all the prostatic tissue. This procedure can be performed as an open surgical procedure or a minimally invasive technique with robotics. The potential side effects of this procedure are urinary incontinence and impotence. Having complete urinary incontinence is rare. There are still a significant number of male patients who will be left with some degree of incontinence and/or impotence following a radical prostatectomy. The extent to which this occurs depends on age, preoperative sexual function, and if the surgery was successful in not injuring the nerves.

Radiation Therapy

There are two types of external beam radiation: photon and proton beam. Photon external beam radiation is the older external radiation therapy. It has several potential side effects. Urinary side effects are common, such as increased urinary frequency and/or painful urination. Erectile dysfunction is seen about one third of the time. The potential gastrointestinal side effects are acute radiation proctitis, abdominal cramping, rectal spasm, urgency of defecation, and long-term diarrhea. Another potential complication from this form of radiation is secondary malignancies, most commonly bladder and rectal cancer. The newer external beam therapy is called a "proton beam radiation therapy." This therapy has a more precise beam to the tumor, with less radiation beam scatter. Because of this there appears to be fewer side effects compared to the photon beam.

Brachytherapy is a direct implantation of a radioactive source into the prostate. This maximizes irradiation of the tumor, while limiting radiation to normal surrounding structures. Permanently implanted seeds of either iodine-125 or palladium-103 are placed into the prostate. This therapy is ideal for men with lower risk disease. This is often used with a prostate cancer that has a PSA less than ten, a Gleason score of less than six, and there are no signs of metastatic disease. Complications associated with this procedure are urinary frequency, urgency, and pain on urination. The risk for erectile dysfunction varies widely and depends on pretreatment condition. Less common is rectal urgency, bleeding, or ulceration. Increased bowel movements and fistulas can also occur.

Androgen (Male Hormone) Deprivation Therapy

This is the preferred initial treatment for men with metastatic prostate cancer. Remember, you cannot give testosterone to a man with prostate cancer because it can accelerate growth. The opposite is also true. If you block testosterone production in the body, you can slow down prostate cancer growth. It can improve quality of life by reducing bone pain as well as rates of complications, such as pathologic fracture, spinal cord compression, and ureteral obstruction. This can be achieved either surgically by castration or medically by various drugs that block the production of testosterone. There are several common side effects associated with this therapy. They include: loss of lean body mass, increased body fat, decreased muscle strength, sexual dysfunction with loss of libido and erectile dysfunction, loss of bone density, hot flashes, gynecomastia (development of male breasts), decreased body hair, fatigue, and smaller penis and testicles.

Choosing the Option of "Watchful Waiting"

These are usually older gentlemen who have been found to have metastatic prostate cancer and there is no hope of cure. They are treated with different forms of palliative care as problems arise. Oncologists will use such modalities as powerful pain medications, androgen deprivation therapy (see above) and radiation therapy for bone pain and nerve compression.

Prostate Cancer Prevention

Unfortunately prostate cancer isn't quite as simple as some cancer in decreasing the risk of developing the disease. To lower your risk of getting lung cancer, for example, a man can refrain from smoking or he can avoid second-hand smoke. Until recently I didn't have a lot to offer my patients to decrease their prostate cancer risk. The good news is recent studies that have shown that by simply improving your lifestyle you may be able to decrease your prostate cancer risk, or at the very least slow down the progression of prostate cancer.

In a study that looked at gentleman who had low-grade prostate cancer, they divided the group into two groups, the experimental group and the control group. The patients in the experimental arm were encouraged to adopt a low-fat, plant-based diet, to exercise and practice stress management, and to attend group support sessions. The control patients received the usual care. After two years 13 of 49 (27 percent) control patients and 2 of 43 (5 percent) experimental patients had undergone conventional prostate cancer treatment (radical prostatectomy, radiotherapy, or androgen deprivation).[47] This was huge difference in disease progression between the two groups. So the factors needed to promote healthy lifestyles such as moderated exercise, mostly a plant based diet and lowering stress, may be a mechanism to decreasing your risk of developing prostate cancer.

12

Brain Health

Can we prevent a decline in mental functions?

More than 35 years ago when I was in medical school, I was taught that by the age of 21 my brain was as big as it was going to be. After that my brain would slowly shrink away, and there was nothing I could do about it. I was told that brain tissue could not regenerate. It was a frightening experience—I was sure I was going to be demented by the age of forty. I was afraid to hold my breath for fear I would lose dozens of brain cells. Fortunately, this theory no longer holds and we now know our brains have some regenerative abilities.

Families often ask me if their family member with memory loss has dementia or Alzheimer's. Dementia is the global term for the loss of mental function to the extent that thinking, memory, and reasoning is severe enough to interfere with a person's daily functioning, whatever the cause. In other words, Alzheimer's is a form of dementia.

I like to divide dementia into two groups: reversible and non-reversible. As a physician, if a patient comes to see me about memory loss—or if an individual comes to discuss a family member with memory loss—I first look for reversible forms of dementia, rather than assuming it a progressive non-reversible dementia. I use this approach even if a person already has been diagnosed with a non-reversible form of dementia, such as Alzheimer's. When I was the medical director of a large nursing home in Cincinnati, Ohio, most of my patients had some severe physical and/or mental disability that prevented them they from caring for themselves. In my care of these nursing home patients, if I had someone who was noted to have a change or worsening in his or her mental status, I would first look for an underlying correctable cause for this decline and not assume that it was due to a progression of the underlying dementia or stroke.

Reversible Dementia

Let's take a look at reversible causes of mental decline. When we reach senior status, we often become isolated. We lose friends, family, and loved ones. The replacement for those losses is sometimes alcohol. I am not saying a person can never have a drink, but what I am saying is that when a person becomes isolated, he often turns to alcohol to cover up the pain of his losses. That five o'clock drink can become the four o'clock, which can become the three o'clock. . . . It is important to know that alcohol can be a neurotoxin. Most of us know people who have consumed excessive amounts of alcohol during their lifetime. Their ability to perform many routine mental activities is often hindered and their reaction time slows down.

Whenever I am doing a workup on a patient looking for causes of nerve injuries to peripheral nerves (these patients often complain of burning and numbness in their feet or hands), I immediately think of two potential culprits for that type of nerve injury. Those two potential neurotoxic elements are diabetes or alcohol. If alcohol can injure our peripheral nerves (nerves that are outside the spinal cord or in the brain), it certainly has the potential for injuring the brain. So if you or a loved one are concerned about drinking in excess, please address the issue and consider professional help, if needed.

Another major source of mental decline is medication. If after being placed on a new drug there appears to be memory problems, the most obvious culprit is the new medication. Some common drug groups that can cause a mental change or decline are pain medications, antidepressants, and seizure medications. In reality, almost any drug has the potential of causing a mental change. In my 30-plus years of practicing medicine, I have seen some of the most harmless drugs cause mental changes. I have seen children and young adults have reciprocal reactions to antihistamines. Most people get tired from the use of the older antihistamines; however, those individuals who have a reciprocal reaction will become hyper-excitable and anxious. The simple answer is, if you start a new medication and there are mental changes, assume that it's the new drug until proven otherwise.

If you are already taking medications and you are placed on a new medicine, you may note a mental change. This can be caused by a drug-drug interaction. The body may be overwhelmed by the additional medication and cannot break down both medications at the same time. When this occurs, toxic levels of the medications may build up. This can be especially true with the elderly. The elderly often have a decreased ability to break down medications due to aging. They are also more likely to be on multiple medications.

As the director of nursing homes, I would complete the initial evaluation on the new patients. It was not unusual for me to see patients who were on more than ten medications. It is no wonder that many of these patients were confused, with all the drug-drug interactions and the decreased ability to metabolize them. On rare occasions I sent some patients home from the nursing home after I was able to slowly wean them off many of their medications. Please note, if you feel you or someone you are caring for is taking too many medications, do not take the self-initiative to suddenly stop them. The action of stopping or weaning off medications needs to be handled under the care of your physician. There are too many potential consequences when suddenly discontinuing medications.

Other correctable medical conditions that can affect mental function are endocrine disorders, such as thyroid disease (both low and high thyroid), parathyroid disease (it can alter calcium levels that can affect your mental functioning), and diabetes with changes in blood sugars. In studies looking at hypothyroidism (low thyroid), the patients were found to have slower reaction times, reduced verbal fluency, and impaired visual memory.[48] By correcting these conditions, mental dysfunction can often be cleared up.

Another cause of reversible mental decline is a topic we will talk more about in the next chapter, and that is sleep disturbances. Good sleep is needed before a memory is formed to organize the memory, and it is also needed after a memory to consolidate the memory. Just improving one's sleep can often correct a person's memory problems.

If a person has a serious illness of a major organ outside of the brain, such as the liver or the kidneys, it can affect one's thinking and memory. The answer to helping these individuals isn't addressing any type of brain dysfunction; it is treating the underlying organ malady.

A final note associated with reversible dementias is sensory deprivation. Many men tend to ignore their declining senses. This can be seen with men who refuse to get their cataracts taken care of or wear hearing aids. With sensory deprivation, a person becomes isolated. To the public these individuals appear to have mental decline since they are unable to follow along in routine conversation. From this isolation there is also the potential of having even more mental decline through depression. Again, we are talking about correctable intellectual impairment. Get the cataracts fixed and wear your hearing aids!

Non-Reversible Dementia

What about those dementias that have a progressive downhill course? These are the non-reversible dementias. The following are a list of those forms of loss of cognitive functions:

- **Alzheimer's:** This is the most common form of the non-reversible dementia. It is seen in 60 to 80 percent of all non-reversible dementias. The microscopic brain tissue of these patients shows two classic findings, and they are called beta amyloid (protein substances that clump to form plaques between the nerve cells in the brain) and neurofibrillary tangles (twisted microtubules resulting from a build up of tau protein inside the nerve cell.)[49] The estimated lifetime risk for men to develop Alzheimer's is 1 in 10.[50]

- **Vascular Dementia:** This is the second most common form of non-reversible dementias; these individuals have multiple small strokes throughout the brain.[51]

- **Lewy Body Dementia:** This is generally associated with individuals who develop dementia that have known Parkinson's disease. What is pathognomonic of these brains is the deposition of another specific protein called Lewy bodies.[52]

- **Pick's Disease:** This dementia is unusual because it starts out as a localized impairment in the brain. A person will begin to have a specific neurologic deficit in one region of the brain. The regions initially affected are usually the temporal and frontal lobes. Over time the dementia will spread globally throughout the brain.

- **Huntington's Dementia:** Huntington's is genetically derived dementia that has an earlier onset than most of the rest of the dementias. The famous songwriter Woody Guthrie suffered from this rapidly progressive loss of cognition.

- **Infectious Dementias:** These are seen in individuals who are suffering with end-stage AIDS. This is a progressive dementia that occurs at the end of their lives. Another infectious type of dementia is Creutzfeldt-Jakob disease. A form of it is called mad cow disease. This is caused by the transfer of tiny protein particles called prions from one person to another or in the case of mad cow disease from cow to human. This protein can be transferred by cutting oneself while working on the brain of an infected cow or person.

- **Chronic Traumatic Encephalopathy:** What occurs with this form of dementia is the deposition of protein particles in the brain called tau proteins, after an individual sustains head traumas. This was discussed in detail in chapter 3.

The question at this point is whether there is anything you can do to prevent these nonreversible dementias. The answer in the past has been generally no, unless you are talking about trauma-induced dementias, in which case you can prevent head traumas by avoiding contact sports or having better rules and regulations in these sports. For the infectious dementias, it means taking as many precautions as possible (wearing condoms to prevent AIDS and double gloving when dealing with the brains of infected individuals or animals with mad cow disease.) The more we understand these diseases, the better we are at learning ways to potentially slow down their progression.

Preventative Measures to Maintain Brain Health

Whenever I give a talk at Canyon Ranch about brain health, I ask my audience to repeat after me and say, "What is good for the heart is good for the brain." In other words, all those things we talked about in the heart chapter that can cause heart disease have the potential for causing brain disease. Those factors include high blood pressure, smoking, diabetes, increased inflammation, and elevated cholesterol. Eliminating these factors is good for your brain. This is especially true with prevention of vascular dementias.

Being physically inactive is another risk factor for intellectual deterioration. The number-one way to decrease the risk of non-reversible dementia is to exercise. The great news is that it is never too late to gain some advantage from exercise. It has been shown that even individuals in their eighties benefited from an exercise program.[53] Other studies have shown that older individuals who participated in aerobic exercises tended to have larger brain volumes of gray and white matter. Shaping and toning, however, did not seem to have an effect on brain volume.[54]

Elevated oxidative stress appears to increase the risk of dementia.[55] A way of measuring oxidative stress was discussed in the heart chapter. This test is called F2 isoprostanes. Certainly if your F2 isoprostanes are high, you need to aggressively lower the level. Having a high oxidative stress means there is an elevated level of free radicals in the body. These are oxidized chemicals in the body that can do some serious damage to your tissues. These nasty "radicals" have the potential of causing significant harm to our more delicate tissue in the body, namely brain tissue.

One of the primary ways to combat free radicals is not to overeat. One of the largest producers of free radicals is food, so eating excessive amounts of food increases free radical production. Another way of decreasing free radicals is to eat those foods that gobble them up, known as antioxidant foods. The capacity of a food to get rid of oxidative stress in the body can be measured. It is called an ORAC (Oxygen Radicle Absorptive Capacity) value. A list of foods can be found on the USDA website: http://www.orac-info-portal.de/download/ORAC_R2.pdf. In viewing this list it is obvious that the best antioxidant foods are berries.[56] I personally make it a point to eat a bowl of berries every day. There are studies that have shown that individuals who drank three to five cups of coffee a day had less dementia.[57] (Coffee is a weak antioxidant. That may be why you need to drink a lot of coffee to get the antioxidant effect).

Finally, meditating may help to prevent mental decline. Studies have revealed that meditating on a regular basis has been shown to have a positive effect in the areas of attention, memory, verbal fluency, and cognitive flexibility.[58]

13

Muscle Function

Problems that can occur with exercise

As I have stated previously, almost everyday I get up in the morning and embark on some form of exercise. I hear my patients all the time telling me that I must exercise because I love to exercise. They say they don't exercise because they hate to exercise or they just don't have time to exercise. Well, I can tell you I don't love to exercise. The greatest part of exercising to me is finishing my exercise. If I go for a run or cycle, I can't wait to get around that last bend in the path because I know I am almost home. As I get older it is getting even more difficult to get myself to exercise because I get stiffer and stiffer every morning. So why do I exercise? The answer is simple. It is one of the best things I can do to keep my body young and healthy.

So what is a good exercise for you? The answer is to find an exercise that you will continue doing on a regular basis. Certainly it is okay to experiment with different types of exercises until you find one that works best for you.

There are three major types of exercise. They are: cardiovascular exercise, weight training, and flexibility training.

Cardiovascular Exercise

I feel cardiovascular exercise is the most important type of exercise that we can do. That is not to say that the other two types (weight training and flexibility training) are unimportant and not good for you. I make this statement because regular cardiovascular exercise has been shown to significantly decrease the risk of chronic diseases such as heart disease, diabetes, cancer, and as is pointed out in chapter 12, may decrease the risk of dementia. For many of us, especially those individuals that struggle to exercise, this is what pushes us to the gym, or the pool or the track. This is the exercise that men will initially gravitate to if they develop one of these diseases and are trying to battle back from them.

Cardiovascular exercise uses large muscle groups in the body to increase the heart rate. With an elevated heart rate there is an increased blood flow throughout the body that will improve oxygenation to the tissues. To maximize the effect of this form of exercise, you have to perform the exercise to a level of intensity that the heart rate will increase to at least 70 percent of its maximum. (A good guesstimate of your heart's maximum heart rate is to take the number 220 minus your age).

There are two forms of cardiovascular exercises. They are aerobic and anaerobic exercises. Aerobic exercises are exercises in which you are able to attain a heart rate of 70 percent of its predicted maximum but not to go above 85 percent of its predicted maximum heart rate. If during your exercise your heart rate does go above the 85 percent predicted it is then considered to be anaerobic. When one at regular intervals during their exercise goes to this anaerobic state, it is called High Intensity Interval Training. Aerobic and anaerobic exercises are discussed in more detail in chapter 16 (pages 175–178). The positive effects from exercise are as follows: aerobic exercise helps keep your weight under control and decreases the risk of developing chronic disease states (heart disease, diabetes, etc.). Intermittently increasing your exercise intensity to an anaerobic state decreases disease risk plus it can increase your fitness. It has also been shown to increase the caloric burn up to two times the rate of aerobic exercises.

For it to be effective you must do a cardiovascular workout a minimum of three days a week for at least 30 minutes to get the positive effects from this exercise.

Weight Training

The prime age for a man to lift weights is during his 20s and 30s. All the men's records in the weight lifting are in this age group. This is the time of maximal muscle strength. The far majority of us are not competing in weight lifting competitions so why should we weight train especially after we have passed our prime? The answer, and it will be discussed more in chapter 15, is that your musculature is where we burn most of the calories we ingest. For this reason our muscle mass is the major source of what makes up our metabolic rate. The more muscles you have, the more the calories you can burn up. The other major reason for weight training, especially as we get older is to give us better stability and balance. Even though our highest capacity for strength is in our 20s and 30s, it does not mean you cannot increase your strength at any time in your life.

There are two basic types of weight training, isotonic and isometric. Isotonic weight training is when a muscle contracts to move some form of weight and there is muscle movement. With isometric weight training there is muscle contraction but no muscle movement. An example of an isotonic exercise is lifting a weight. An example of an isometric exercise is standing in a doorway and pushing with both arms against the door jams. If you are not the Hulk, muscle contraction will take place but there will no movement of the door jam. Both isotonic and isometric exercises can be used to develop strength, muscle size, and muscular endurance; however, isotonic exercises are generally better for increasing functional strength compared to isometric exercises.[59]

- **Isotonic exercise:** This kind of exercise has two phases. Concentric contraction is when the muscle contracts to lift or pull a weight. The muscle shortens causing the joint angle to decrease. The next phase called eccentric contraction is when the muscle lengthens and there is an increase in the joint angle. During isotonic exercises muscle groups are isolated to increase strength and improve performance. To do effective weight training you should do 2 to 3 sets of 8 to 12 reps with the major muscle groups two to three times a week. The major muscle groups include your hamstrings, quadriceps, calves, butt, back, chest, shoulders, biceps, triceps, and abdominal muscles.[60]

- **Isometric weight lifting:** Strength adaptations from isometric exercise are a function of the length of time the body is held in position. You need to contract the muscle and hold that position for as long as possible until you have muscle failure and fatigue. Isometric exercise is an excellent form of weight training for your core body muscles. By strengthening these muscles it has been shown to stabilize your spine. This can be helpful if you have any kind of chronic back pain.

One particular isometric exercise that strengthens your core muscles is the yoga plank position. To accomplish this exercise start on your hands and knees with your wrists directly under your shoulders. Draw your abdominal muscles toward your spine. Next tuck your toes and step back and bring your body and head into a straight line. Remain in this straight line for as long as you can maintain it. Hopefully, over time you will be able to stay in this position for over one minute.

It is important to know that isometric exercises can cause a rise in a person's blood pressure. For that reason I do not advise doing isometric exercises if you have uncontrolled high blood pressure.

Another group of individuals that we don't always think about promoting weight lifting to are those individuals that may have suffered a major illness. With the disability that can occur with a major illness, there can be a significant amount of muscle wasting. This has the potential to increase the risk of premature mortality, injurious falls, bone fracture, and disability. In a study that looked at cancer survivors, there was a 50 percent decrease in muscle wasting in the group that performed a slowly progressive weight lifting program compared with standard care.[61]

Stretching Exercise

There are several advantages to stretching: It can decrease injuries, it can help relieve musculoskeletal pain that is seen with arthritis, fibromyalgia, and chronic back pain. It is also helpful in improving balance, flexibility, and coordination. It is important to stretch not only before any other kind of exercising, but also to stretch immediately after exercising when your muscles are already heated up. One can focus on stretching by doing such practices as yoga. It appears that most athletes show some benefit from yoga. The only problem that may occur is if one develops excessive flexibility with advanced yoga. Some athletic performances can be hindered in their performance if this occurs. (For the far majority of us this is rarely a problem, especially if we do yoga less than three times a week.)[62] Some very basic stretching exercises are demonstrated on pages 8, 9, 10, and 11 of the photo insert.

Muscle Injuries and Heat-Related Disorders

Exercised-induced Muscle Cramps

This is very common to anyone who exercises. It is commonly seen in those individuals who are starting to exercise or are increasing their duration or intensity of their present exercise program. Muscle cramps can be a very painful experience. In high school I remember that every summer during the first week of football practice, I was awakened in the middle of the night with severe muscle spasms in my calves. My screams would wake everyone in the house, and my dad would have to come to my bedroom and rub my legs until the cramps went away.

For years it has been thought that these cramps were due to dehydration and electrolyte imbalance from excessive sweating while exercising. This is part of the problem, but it is now felt to be more complicated than that. There appears to be an element of muscle fatigue from overuse of the muscles, which can affect the tendons and nerves of the reflex arch. The treatment is rehydration, replacements of electrolytes, and rest. (The electrolyte solutions can be obtained from good running or cycling stores. One of the more respected companies is called Hammer, which makes a sports powder to be mixed with water called HEED.) In addition, routine stretching exercises should be done. The stretch needs to be done in such a way that the muscle needs to be slowly lengthened until the muscle spasm or excess tightness is deactivated.

DOMS—Delayed Onset Muscle Soreness

This is different than the more common exercise induced muscle cramps. It will occur late in an exercise program or an athletic event. This will develop one or two days after the exercise. With this process there is actual damage to the muscle cells and an inflammatory reaction occurs in the muscles.[63] DOMS can be seen in an elite athlete or the beginning exerciser. The symptoms are severe muscular pain and muscle tenderness. It is seen most commonly at the beginning of the sporting season or when someone starts an exercise program. Treatment consists of rest, using non-steroidal anti-inflammatory agents (like ibuprofen), and massage. Cryotherapy, ultrasound, stretching, and electrical stimulation have not proved to be effective. Novel activities should be introduced progressively over a period of one or two weeks at the beginning of, or during, the sporting season in order to reduce the risk of developing this syndrome.

Heat Exhaustion

This is when the body still has the capability to thermoregulate, but it has been overwhelmed by excessive heat and can't get rid of it. During heat exhaustion the body's temperature is below 39 degrees C (102.2 degrees). These individuals will complain of feeling extreme fatigue, and feeling lightheaded. They will demonstrate shortness of breath and have a rapid pulse and low blood pressure. Their skin may be hot and dry. The usual culprit is that the individual has lost excessive amounts of fluids and electrolytes from exercise. Individuals that are out of shape and not acclimated to the outside heat are the most susceptible to this problem.

The treatment is electrolyte fluids, either given orally if the person is conscious and able to keep fluids down, or given intravenously if not. To prevent this problem, keep up with your liquids as you exercise. When exercising less than an hour, drink plenty of water before, during, and after exercising. Your urine should always be clear or light yellow. If it gets darker than that, you are not drinking enough. Whenever exercising longer than one hour, it is important to drink electrolyte solutions that can replace the salts that are being lost from sweating.

Heat Stroke

This is a life-threatening emergency. If not addressed rapidly, the person can progress to a coma and then death. Once again these individuals become dehydrated; they lose excessive electrolytes, but what is different from heat exhaustion, is that these individuals lose the ability to thermoregulate.

These victims have the following signs and symptoms:

- Their body temperature is > 40 degrees C (104.9 degrees F)
- The skin is hot and dry
- They quit sweating
- They have an altered consciousness
- Blood pressure is often elevated
- They have a rapid weak pulse

These individuals need to be rapidly cooled and be given IV fluids. Once again, this is an emergency situation and must be treated as such; otherwise death may ensue.

When I see a patient, unless they are physical unable to do so, one of my most nonnegotiable prescriptions that I give to them is they must do some form of exercise program. I have no better drug to offer them for their health and well-being. I encourage them, and I encourage you, the reader, to have a regular routine of a cardiovascular exercise at least three times a week, to weight train a minimum of two days a week, and to do some form of stretching almost daily. It is important to know that there is a higher risk of muscle injures as you start your exercise program and finally be sure to be well hydrated before, during, and after you exercise.

Your Health by Strategy

14

Sleep Better

Sleeping is more powerful than you think.

Sorry guys, but whether you receive a bad rap or not, many of you are implicated in doing a lot of snoring and accused by partners of giving them a miserable night. The result of all this snoring is poor quality of sleep for both you and your bed partner.

We can't ignore the numbers. Sleep disorders are seen more commonly in men than women, and snoring is just one of the many types of sleeping problems. It is very important to recognize when a person has a condition that causes sleep disturbance. Untreated sleep problems increase the risk for multiple health issues, including hypertension, diabetes, obesity, and heart disease.

The majority of my male patients with sleep disorders do not make an appointment to see me because they think they have a problem with their sleep. They come because their partner sent them. The person sharing their bed is either frustrated by the incessant snoring and being kicked all night, or if my patient has been diagnosed with sleep apnea, their partner is worried sick when he periodically stops breathing and spends the night anxiously listening to make sure he's resumed breathing again.

Men tend to feel that being in bed for six or seven hours constitutes a good night's sleep. They do not realize that the quality of sleep can be as important as the quantity. My patient Jim was a classic example of this. He never thought he had a problem with his sleep, but his wife kept insisting that he snored and had intermittent episodes of gasping for air while asleep. He kept putting off seeing someone because he thought it was all a bunch of baloney. Fortunately, while on vacation at Canyon Ranch, Jim found out we had a sleep lab at our facility. He finally relented and consented to come in and see me for a consultation. His primary symptom was daytime drowsiness, especially in the early afternoon. He would fall asleep during long meetings, and he could never drive two hours straight without drinking coffee or stopping for a rest. He thought that was normal for everyone.

I advised him to have an overnight split sleep study. The split study means that during Jim's sleep, if he had episodes of obstructive sleep disturbance like those caused by sleep apnea, a sleep technician could attach a CPAP (which stands for continuous positive airway pressure) machine to him. This machine has a mask that covers the face and provides continuous air pressure that keeps the airway open and doesn't allow it to collapse. The technician then monitors the patient from the next room to see if the machine corrected the problem. Jim had wires attached to his head to obtain a continuous brain wave study (called an EEG), and wires were attached to his chest to obtain a continuous EKG. An oxygen sensor was attached to his finger and another sensor was connected to his legs to check to see if he had any excessive leg movement during the night.

During Jim's study the sleep technician noted that Jim had episodes where he stopped breathing and his oxygen levels dropped. For this reason the sleep technician attached the CPAP machine to him. After being connected to the machine, his oxygen levels rose and his disturbed sleep significantly improved. It was decided after the test that Jim needed a CPAP machine. He reluctantly consented, and I sent him home with a machine. I followed Jim's progress over the next six months. His borderline elevated blood pressure resolved, and he was able to lose twenty pounds. Finally, Jim realized he no longer became tired while driving, and he no longer feared falling asleep during long distance driving.

Many people believe that you have to be overweight to have a sleep disturbance. It is true that the incidence of sleep disturbances increases when you are overweight; however, I personally am an example of someone who has a normal weight and still has a sleeping problem. I used to have significant daytime drowsiness. I couldn't make the two-hour drive from Tucson to Phoenix without having to pull over halfway through the trip to rest or get some caffeine. I had a sleep study and was found to have multiple nighttime arousals that I didn't know about. In other words, I didn't actually wake up at night, but I was unable to get deep restorative sleep because of my disturbed sleep. I too needed to be placed on a CPAP machine. After only a few days, I was amazed by my daytime alertness. I no longer worry about those long drives or falling asleep during important meetings.

An easy first step to determine if you have a sleep disturbance is to take the following test called the **Epworth Sleepiness Scale**.[64] A total score of 8 or higher is considered a positive score and means you may have a sleep disturbance. If this is the case you should discuss it with your doctor.

If you do have a sleep problem, please do not ignore it. As I stated previously, poor sleep is a major cause (or a contributing factor) of many severe medical problems. These conditions include heart disease, such as heart failure, cardiac rhythm disturbances, and hypertension. Lack of sleep has been shown to cause weight gain.[65] It is a major culprit in the causes of obesity. With the increased risk of weight gain, there is an increased risk for diabetes. I firmly believe that obtaining good restorative sleep is so crucial for your health that it is a routine part of my history taking during my patients' office visits.

0 = *no chance of dozing*

1 = *slight chance of dozing*

2 = *moderate chance of dozing*

3 = *high chance of dozing*

Situation	Chance of Dozing
Sitting and reading	
Watching TV	
Sitting inactive in a public place (e.g. a theater or a meeting)	
As a passenger in a car for an hour without a break	
Lying down to rest in the afternoon when circumstances permit	
Sitting and talking to someone	
Sitting quietly after a lunch without alcohol	
In a car, while stopped for a few minutes in traffic	

I must admit my eyes were opened to the possible benefits of using sleep medicine after coming to Canyon Ranch. I have been blessed to have worked with two sleep specialists, Dr. Phil Eichling and Dr. Param Dedhia. They have taught me all the different ways in which poor sleep affects our health. It was a standing joke with the medical staff that no matter what kind of medical problem was discussed, Dr. Eichling could relate that problem to some form of sleep problem. More often than not he was right.

Common Sleep Problems

When most people think of sleep disturbances they think of either insomnia, which is when an individual has a hard time falling or remaining asleep, or sleep apnea, which is episodic cessation of breathing. There are actually several different types of sleep problems. Some are very complex and require involvement of medical specialists to diagnose and recommend effective treatments.

Below are the most prevalent in the United States.

Nature of Sleep Disturbances	Who is Affected
Inadequate Sleep	Most of us
"Phase" Disorder (the time for getting up and going to bed is shifted) • Delayed—(common to teens) • Advanced—(common in the elderly)	25 percent of the population 25 percent of the population
Insomnia (can't fall or stay asleep)	10–15 percent of the population
Sleep Apnea (stop breathing) and Snoring	5–10 percent of the population
Nocturnal Movement Disorder	5–10 percent of the population
Narcolepsy (spontaneously falling asleep)	1 in 2,000

The most common type of sleep disturbance is insomnia. Insomnia is defined as a disorder characterized by a difficulty in falling and/or staying asleep. Individuals who suffer from this problem often have hyperactive brains.

Factors that may affect initiation of sleep are a background of anxiety and depression, a condition of chronic pain, and a diagnosis of bipolar disease.

Helpful Strategies for Reducing Insomnia

- Meditate at bedtime. (you can go to https://www.facebook.com/TheCanyonRanchGuidetoMensHealth/ to view a short video on focused meditation))
- Do progressive muscular relaxation (see exercise on pages 12, 13, 14, 15, and 16 of the photo insert).
- Make sure your home is secure and safe.
- Keep the bedroom dark (this may include covering small lights from electronics).
- Turn your clock around so you can't see it.
- Develop a routine prior to going to bed.
- Don't eat, drink, or exercise in late evening.
- If you are in bed for twenty minutes and you can't fall asleep, get up and do something until you are tired.

By following some of these helpful hints, you will often get significant improvement in your nighttime sleep.

I hope reading this chapter has convinced you of the importance of having good sleep. Please don't follow the typical male response and ignore the concerns of your bed partner about abnormal sleep. And please find out where you fall on the Epworth Sleepiness Scale if you have fatigue during the day. Daytime drowsiness is not normal!

15

Nutrition for a Healthy Man

What should real men eat?

As I was developing my chapter on nutrition, I thought about how men and women often eat differently. Guys tend to be carnivores (meat eaters) and women tend to be herbivores (plant eaters). Men love their protein and women tend to love their chocolate. Yes, these are generalities, but after being on this planet for more than sixty years, I haven't seen this basic premise change much.

Studies have shown that women are more likely than men to eat a diet high in fruits and fiber. Women also avoid eating high-fat foods, and they tend to limit their salt intake more than men. This was seen in almost all of twenty-three countries that studied this. Women were more likely to diet and attached greater importance to healthy eating. Gender differences in food choices appear to be partly attributable to women's greater weight control involvement and partly due to their stronger beliefs in healthy eating.[66]

Now that it has been shown that men and women do appear to eat differently, the real question is, should they? Looking at this question from a healthy eating perspective, I feel there are many aspects of our diets in which men and women can and should eat the same and there are parts of the diet in which they may eat differently. The first and most obvious difference between what men and women eat is the amount. Men are generally bigger than women and for that reason need to consume more calories. For those individuals who lead sedentary lifestyles, they should eat about thirteen calories per pound of body weight. Those who engage in moderate exercise need sixteen calories per pound of body weight, and those who exercise vigorously should eat eighteen calories per pound. A more accurate way of looking at this is to visit the following website and enter your numbers: http://nutrition.about.com/library/bl_nutrition_guide_men.htm. It bases the amount of calories you need to eat per day on weight, height, desired weight, and amount of exercise.

Protein

Protein is used to form structural parts of our bodies and is also important for the formation of our enzymes, hormones, and neurotransmitters. There is a misconception among most men that they need to eat a lot of protein especially compared to women. Actually, the National Institutes of Health feels that men only need two to three servings of protein-rich foods daily (https://www.nlm.nih.gov/medlineplus/ency/article/002467.htm). The following are recommended serving sizes for protein: two to three ounces of cooked lean meat, poultry, or fish (a portion is about the size of a deck of playing cards), 1/2 cup of cooked dried beans, 1 egg, 2 tablespoons of peanut butter, or 1 ounce of cheese. To calculate the exact amount of protein required each day can be complicated and you may need the assistance of a nutritionist to be more precise. My point here is that men generally eat more protein than they actually need and the usage of high protein drinks and shakes is rarely warranted. In fact, excess protein in the body increases the amount of calcium loss in the urine, which can increase the risk of osteoporosis and kidney stones.

As a whole, men eat more red meat than women. Well, gentlemen, start thinking twice about it. Unfortunately for you bloody-red meat eaters, the numbers are stacked up against you. When I read now about all the harmful effects that are associated with red meat, I have to shake my head. Growing up the son of a country veterinarian, more than 90 percent of our evening meals were some form of red meat. Every year my father would go to his favorite farmer and buy a whole cow and have it butchered. We had enough beef in our freezer to last for almost an entire year. Every morning my dad would go down to the basement, open the freezer, and pick out what form of beef we would have for dinner that night. He would set the frozen meat out on the kitchen countertop (we now know that was a bad choice) and let it thaw out. When Dad returned home in the evening from working out on the farms, he would cook the evening meal with whatever meat he had set out in the morning. Steaks were our Saturday night special treat. On Sundays we always had some type of pot roast.

So what are the ill effects of red meat? A study published online in March 2012 in the Archives of Internal Medicine suggests that people with higher intakes of red meat faced an increased risk of death.[67] The good news is that if you replace the red meat with healthy proteins, such as fish, poultry, nuts, or legumes, the risk of death decreases. A major culprit in the ill effects of red meat (which includes beef, pork, and lamb) is the high content of saturated fats. This has been shown to increase the risk of cardiovascular disease. My father, my father's brother and sister, and his father all died of a stroke. They all came from the farm in which red meat was their staple. This background has certainly influenced my decision to significantly decrease my consumption of red meats.

At the time I was writing this book, Dr. Stan Hazen, who is the head of research at the Lehrner Center at Cleveland Clinic, found out that there was another chemical in red meat that may also be associated with coronary artery disease. That chemical, L-Carnitine, is found in red meat. In the small intestines L-Carnitine is transformed by the bacteria into a chemical called TMAO (trimethylamine-N-oxide), which promotes atherosclerosis (hardening of the arteries).[68]

Another concern with red meat and processed meat (bacon, hot dogs, cold cuts, and sausages) intake is cancer. These meats have been associated with colon, lung, esophageal, and stomach cancers. Everyone struggles with defining what is a harmful amount. The World Cancer Research Fund, which looks at worldwide environmental impacts on cancer, recommends everyone to eat fewer than eleven ounces of red meat per week.

There is some limited evidence that milk and dairy products increase the risk of prostate cancer.[69] The mechanism could be related to the calcium consumption in the milk and dairy products. High calcium intake may decrease the formation of 1, 25-dihydroxy vitamin D. This has the potential of increasing cell proliferation in the prostate. There are other studies showing that it may not be the calcium in the dairy products that increases this risk of prostate cancer but it may be the dairy proteins consumed. This was pointed out in Dr. Colin Campbell's book *The China Study*. It showed that the amount of dairy protein ingested can reach a critical level, over which there is an increased prostate cancer risk. I personally have lowered my dairy consumption since these reports have been made public. I have not advised elimination of dairy foods, but I have recommended decreasing the quantity of them.

To Juice or Nor to Juice?

Men often ask me if they should juice their foods. Juicing is good, but not the best way to receive good nutrients. Whole foods are always the first choice when it comes to healthy eating. Juicing may contain higher sugar content and generally less fiber. This can increase insulin levels and caloric intake. It may also lack some of the essential nutrients that you can get from whole foods. If you are not going to make the juice yourself, be sure to read labels. Juices can be high in sodium. Store-bought juices often add sugar, so be sure to buy only 100 percent juice.

The best argument for juicing is that it allows a person to eat on the run. Juicing is a convenient way of getting some of the nutrients from fruits and vegetables. It's obviously much quicker to drink a glass of juice than peeling and cutting up fruit or cooking some vegetables. The bottom line is that it is much better to drink a fruit or vegetable juice than not eat any fruits or vegetables at all.

One last piece on juicing is that if you are trying to lose weight, juicing may not always be the best option. It takes energy to digest food. It is called the thermal effect of eating. What this means is that you burn calories when you digest food. It takes energy and calories to chew food then to churn the food and digest the food before you can absorb it. When you juice your food, much of the mechanics of digestion are eliminated and you may not burn as many calories when you eat. This can add to the difficulty in trying to lose weight.

Turning "Almost" Vegetarian and Why You Should Consider It

I am frequently amazed at how my own eating habits have changed over the years. My habits are based on what has been observed in the scientific literature and what I have heard from researchers who have conducted studies on health and diets. I recently listened to a Grand Rounds lecture from the Mayo Clinic in Scottsdale. The lecturer was Dr. Caldwell Esselstyne. He had been a general surgeon at the Cleveland Clinic who, after many years of practicing surgery, decided to turn in his scalpel and change his interest from the operating suite to preventative medicine. His focus was on how to prevent and possibly reverse coronary artery disease. His treatment was not taking high dose statins (cholesterol lowering medications); it was eating a plant-based diet and exercising. Because of this talk and my personal interest in this problem, I decided to look more closely at atherosclerotic disease and diet.

As I stated previously, my father died of a stroke at the age of seventy, my uncle died of a stroke at the age of sixty-two, my aunt died of a stroke in her early seventies, and my grandfather suffered a major stroke in his mid-seventies. All these relatives loved their meats. They were all born and raised on the farm. Their staple food was meat coated with plenty of gravy. Breakfast started with eggs, bacon, and sausage. Lunchtime was cold meat sandwiches, and dinner was some type of beef as the main course. This carried on with their children (that's me!). We loved to eat meat, especially red meat. So here we go again with another generation of plaque formers! My family could easily be its own little scientific study on atherosclerotic disease.

Prior to Dr. Caldwell Esselstyne's talk, I had learned that a near vegetarian diet, along with other associated lifestyle changes, had made an improvement on coronary artery plaque. For several years I had already decreased my consumption of all meats, especially red meats. Some of the early work in looking at a decreased meat intake was first published by Dean Ornish in the 1990s.[70] When I first read Dr. Ornish's work, I was seeing a very small number of patients and was told by many who attempted this diet that it was difficult to maintain. However, after listening to Dr. Esselstyne lecture, I had an epiphany. If I have plaque formation, I have the ability to decrease it by changing to a more plant-based diet.

Dr. T. Colin Campbell has also found a correlation with animal-based diets and the risk of cancers. (Both Caldwell Esselstyne and T. Colin Campbell were the focus of the excellent documentary *Forks over Knives*.) Not only do I personally have a family history of vascular disease but also I have a strong family history of cancers with both my grandmother and aunt dying of cancer. With this double-edged sword of a family history staring me down, I finally decided to become almost vegan. I now feel better overall and have more energy than I have had in a long time.

The number one question that men ask about a vegetarian diet is how can they get enough protein in their diet if they don't eat meat. The answer is that there are plenty of plant-based choices to obtain protein. This can be seen with beans, such as black beans, kidney beans, pinto beans, and garbanzo beans. Other good sources of protein are from lentil, split peas, and nuts and seeds including almonds, hazelnuts, mixed nuts, peanuts, peanut butter, sunflower seeds, or walnuts; and another good source are soy products like tofu. Grains are also great sources of protein, and they can include buckwheat, oats, rye, millet, maize (corn), rice, wheat, bulgur, sorghum, amaranth, and quinoa. Protein is found in all whole plant foods, and it has not been demonstrated that we require more than what is found naturally in a varied whole-food, plant-based diet that is sufficient in calories.

No, I haven't gone over the deep end on this one. Healthy living is a continuum. Some people feel improving their diet is simply cutting down the amount of fried food they eat. Others may feel that decreasing the amount of red meat they eat per week from six days a week to three days a week is a vast improvement. For them, it may be true. I am giving what appears to be, at this time, the best diet when it comes to prevention of chronic illness. These diseases include coronary artery disease, strokes, cancers, and diabetes.

As I said, healthy eating, like all forms of healthy behavior, is a continuum and does not have to be an all or nothing phenomenon. The closer we are to attaining a healthy diet, the healthier we can generally be. Certainly an individual who eats red meat six days a week, stuffs down plenty of deep fried food, and calls ketchup his daily vegetable is generally in much worse condition than someone who eats red meat twice a week, avoids fried food, and eats two servings of vegetables a day.

It's amazing that once people start improving their diet, they often will continue to improve it until they reach a point where they feel they have gone as far as they think they can go and will stay at that level for some time. After a finite period of time, these individuals may improve their diet even more. As they start to feel better, they might find out that brussels sprouts actually taste good. I am not here to tell you how perfect your diet should be. I am simply giving you choices on your own personal continuum to better health.

So what is my recommendation to the reader? I feel at this point there is strong evidence that red meat is not good for you, and the less you eat the better. Other animal proteins should be limited. We all have to find out what we are comfortable with in either decreasing or eliminating meats. Certainly, if there is a strong family history of cardiovascular disease in relationship to plaque build-up, or there is a family history of cancers, then you should consider eating closer to a vegan type of diet.

If you would decide to "go all the way" and eat a vegetarian diet, there is one nutrient that is missing and must be replaced. That nutrient is Vitamin B12. You will need to take at least one hundred micrograms a day of this supplement daily.

Vitamins, Minerals, and Supplements

In looking at vitamins and minerals, there are two very different requirements for men and women. The first is iron. Men don't need as much iron as a menstruating female. The requirement for men is no more than eight milligrams a day. Men also need much less calcium than women. Excessive amounts can lead to kidney stones. There is some question as to whether calcium supplementation in men may increase the risk of prostate cancer.[71] There is also a concern regarding calcium supplementation and the potential of calcium deposition in the arteries, which may contribute to atherosclerosis. These have been conflicting studies, but I do not routinely recommend calcium supplementation for my male patients.

It has been my experience that women take more supplements than men. I often hear from men that they take the vitamins and supplements that their wives have set out for them. Overall, my opinion about supplements has changed since writing my last book. My recommendation for their use has significantly decreased. Supplements need to be exactly what the name implies—they should "supplement" the nutrients that we may lack in our diets or are not receiving from the environment. Two examples are vitamin D and B12. Vitamin D is needed if you live in a sun-deprived environment like Seattle. To obtain vitamin D naturally, our skin needs exposure to the sun. And as we just discussed, if you are a vegetarian, you will need supplemental vitamin B12.

I am often asked by patients what supplements they should take. Some are already taking supplements and just want to know if they should take more. Others are considering taking supplements, because their friends are taking them or their personal trainer says they need to be taking them for their health. My bottom line is that the usage of supplements is always individualized. It is the proverbial "one shoe does not fit all." There is so much variation in a person's diet and his physical workloads that an individual approach is always the best.

Generally, I would like to have the patient discuss supplements and vitamins with their family physician. Hopefully, you can work with a practitioner who can evaluate your blood chemistries and your diet and who knows your genetics and your personality, and then can direct you to the appropriate supplements and vitamins, if needed. If you don't have access to a knowledgeable doctor who understands the world of supplements and vitamins, then I have a few general suggestions.

Omega-3 Fish Oils

I feel men should consider taking fish oil supplement if they are not eating at least two fish meals a week. More recent studies have not been as convincing about the advantages of omega-3 fish oils in the prevention of heart disease as earlier studies, but overall they still seem to have a benefit. The older articles written showed significant benefit in the prevention of heart disease with omega-3 fish oils; however, the newer articles are written when people have made other lifestyle changes that have lowered the overall risk of heart disease. Also, the newer trials used lower-dose omega-3s and compared them to relatively high-baseline omega-3s. The American Heart Association still recommends 1 gram of EPA/DHA for patients with coronary heart disease.[72] Exceptions are made to this recommendation of taking fish oils if you are a vegetarian, you are allergic to fish oil, or you have a bleeding tendency.

During the time of the writing of this book, there was a paper that appeared to show a correlation between prostate cancer and the level of omega-3 fatty acids. Higher levels of omega-3s seem to have a higher incidence of prostate cancer.[73] This has not been reproduced and it was not a prospective study. (A prospective study would have started with two groups of men without prostate cancer and gave one group of high-level omega-3s and another group of low omega-3s to see which group developed more prostate cancer.) It generally has been disputed among the medical establishment, and for that reason I continue to recommend fish oils unless there is a strong family history of prostate cancer, and then it should be a discussion between you and your doctor about the risk benefits before a decision is made.

When buying omega-3 fish oils be sure to get enough of the right type of omega-3s. Try to get around one thousand milligrams of EPA and DHA total per day.

Vitamin D

Over the past few years, vitamin D has received a lot of press. It is not the cure-all for whatever ails you, but it is important for many aspects of our health, especially bone health. When I was growing up, my mother told us to go outside and "get some sun." There was never a mention about using suntan lotion. Since that time the medical field has asked the public to stay out of the sun as much as possible, because they determined that the number one cause of skin cancers was exposure to the sun. If a person needed to be out in the sun, he was told to shield his skin with protective clothing and wear suntan lotion. These maneuvers were helpful in decreasing the incidence of skin cancers. Unfortunately, little sun exposure has led to a populous that is low in vitamin D.

Our basic source for vitamin D is the sun. When the sun hits our skin with ultraviolet light, it converts 7-hydroxycholesterol into vitamin D_3. Vitamin D_3 then travels to the liver and is converted to 25-OH hydroxyvitamin D that goes to the kidney and is converted to 1,25-OH dihydroxyvitamin D. It is this last chemical that helps increase calcium absorption from the gut and it decreases calcium loss from the kidneys. Having calcium available is essential for building healthy bone.

There are other potential usages for vitamin D. It has been shown to be helpful in preventing falls in older people, and it helps reduce bone loss in people taking drugs called corticosteroids.

Vitamin D "may" (and I am using this term loosely) be helpful in the following:

- Decreasing the risk of multiple sclerosis (MS). We know that the higher in latitude someone lives (in the northern hemisphere), the incidence of multiple sclerosis is increased. The farther north one lives, the less sunlight they will receive.

- Preventing cancer. This is a big statement. Some preliminary studies suggest this. We will need to see more studies to see if this holds up.

- Respiratory infections. Taking a vitamin D supplement during winter may reduce the chance of getting seasonal flu.
- Preventing tooth loss in the elderly.

There are many other potential benefits that have been proclaimed about vitamin D. These include helping depression (especially seasonal effective disorder that is related to decreased sunlight), treating diabetes, and preventing heart disease. More studies need to be conducted before all these "other benefits" are confirmed.

Often one of the first signs that a man may have low vitamin D is if he is found to have a low bone density. This raises an important point. I feel men need to have their bone density checked. Women commonly have this done but men usually ignore it. I recommend that men start having a bone density study done at the age of 50. If a man's bone density reveals signs of bone loss, one of the first things I do is obtain a vitamin D blood level. My personal recommendation is to have a 25-OH hydroxyvitamin D blood level greater than 30 nanograms/milliliter. The upper level has been controversial. At this time, I don't want that level to be greater than 60 nanograms per milliliter (many reference ranges will say that the upper limits are as high as 100 nanograms per milliliter).

It needs to be noted that problems can occur if you take too much vitamin D. Do not fall into that All-American trap that if a little is good then more is better. With too much vitamin D, you can get excessive calcium levels in the body that can deposit in your soft tissues and in other organs. Calcium deposition in the kidneys can lead to kidney failure. Because your blood level is important, I recommend obtaining a vitamin D blood level (25-OH vitamin D blood level) before you start taking vitamin D to first determine if you need a vitamin D supplement. If you start taking a vitamin D supplement, I then advise you to recheck your vitamin D level one month later to determine if you are taking the proper amount.

In general, if your blood level shows you are mildly deficient in vitamin D, 20 to 30 nanograms per milliliter, then I would have you start at 1000 IU of vitamin D$_3$ daily. If it is less than 20 nanograms per milliliter, I would have you start at 2,000 IU of vitamin D$_3$ daily. Once again, if you decide to take a vitamin D supplement, please follow up with a blood test through your family doctor to be sure you are taking the right amount.

The Importance of Gut Health

Men unfortunately assume that bloating and gas are simply part of being a guy. I usually have to ask men if they have any digestive problems and ask specific questions about any problems, explaining what is normal and what isn't. For this reason there are a lot of men out there with a lot of digestive issues who never really address them. So why look into something that doesn't seem like a real problem? The answer is twofold. First, why suffer discomfort if you don't have to? Second, this discomfort and bloating may indicate poor digestion, which can affect your health.

We need to not only eat nutritious foods but also we need to effectively absorb those foods. The steps to a normal healthy food absorption start with a mechanical and chemical digestion of food. Next, the digested foods must be moved across the intestinal wall to be absorbed into the blood stream. Poor absorption of nutrients into the body is called malabsorption. There are many different causes of malabsorption. You can be born with an absorptive problem or you can acquire one. Most of the congenital (born with abnormality) forms of malabsorption are varied and for the most part rare. We will therefore only discuss the more common acquired forms.

The mechanical portion of digestion is accomplished by the churning action of the stomach. An abnormal or decreased movement by the stomach is called gastroparesis, and it results in delayed stomach emptying. Estimates reveal that 20 to 40 percent of patients with diabetes, primarily those with long duration type 1 diabetes mellitus, will have this problem. This can cause a lot of abdominal distress, because the food is not moved through the GI tract.

The chemical digestion occurs initially from hydrochloric acid produced by the stomach. As we get older the production of acid decreases. A common self-induced way to decrease acid production is by the usage of one of the multiple drugs designed to decrease acid secretion. These medications are the H2 blockers, like Zantac and Pepcid and the proton pump inhibitors like Prilosec or Nexium. Many of us suffer from a syndrome called gastroesophageal reflux, which responds to these over-the-counter medications, decreasing the burning in our chests after eating.

Initially, they do help us feel better. The problem is that we produce acid for a reason; it is the beginning of the chemical breakdown of food. All these acid reducer medications have created poor digestion. Food often isn't broken down as well with the reduced production of acid, and therefore it remains in the gut longer because it can't be absorbed as well. This can cause abdominal discomfort. (It should be noted that another serious condition that results from taking excessive use of these medications is osteoporosis.[74] This stems from a decreased ability to break down and absorb the minerals used to make healthy bone.)

When appropriately used, the H2 blockers and proton pump inhibitors are worth their weight in gold—there is no question reflux can be a miserable experience. Not only can reflux cause symptomatic problems with the burning sensation but also, if left untreated, it can lead to serious problems, such as inflammation in the esophagus called esophagitis. When I was in medical school, antacids were the only treatment for excess acid secretion. I used to be up all night with patients who had life-threatening bleeding ulcers.

When the first H2 blocker, Tagamet, became available, I suddenly was able to sleep at night. Because of this drug and similar drugs later developed, I know firsthand the impact and the importance of these drugs. With the symptom relief these drugs provide (H2 blockers, or proton pump inhibitors), physicians often encourage their patients to remain on these drugs and never cease using them. However, with prolonged use of these medications and subsequent decreased ability to digest foods, the end result may be bloating and increased gas.

My approach to gastric acid reflux is first to encourage the use of the H2 blockers or proton pump inhibitors to essentially put out the fire. The patients think you are their life savior because the burning finally goes away. I have my patients take these drugs for one to two months. At the same time I prescribe these medications, I will also look for potential causes of the reflux and try to eliminate them. I have told my patients for years that the bad habits that can cause reflux are like the fuel that feeds the fire, and taking the medications is the water that helps put out the fire. It is only common sense that turning off the fuel that feeds the fire is the first real answer, but after that you need to get to the heart of why you have the reflux.

The factors that can cause reflux are alcohol, caffeine, smoking, being overweight, and eating late (especially right before going to bed). Removing these causes of reflux may eliminate the need for medication. My experience has been that men are more likely to continue their poor lifestyles instead of correcting them. They would rather take a simple little pill than correct their bad habits. If they select the pill instead of making lifestyle changes, in the end, they often pay the price with bloating, gassiness, and less than optimal absorption of their nutrients.

Another problem that can occur with the initial phase of digestion is a lack of pancreatic enzymes. These enzymes help break down proteins and fats. The people who are most susceptible to this problem are those with a past history of pancreatitis. These individuals often have a lot of scarring in the pancreas, which causes a decreased production of enzymes. This leads to poor digestion and malabsorption. Aging is another cause of decreased enzymatic production. The classic symptoms are bloating and cramping, which occur in the abdomen about an hour after eating. If you have these symptoms—especially if you have a past history of pancreatitis—ask your pharmacist or doctor about a trial of using pancreatic enzymes. The best time to take the enzymes is with your meals. It is certainly a situation of trial and error. There is little harm that will occur if this does not work, but your life can improve dramatically if it does work.

Other causes of poor digestion can occur when there is damage to the lining of the gut, most notably the small intestines. One of the most severe forms of this digestive problem is a malady called celiac disease. In 1888 Samuel Gee was one of the first individuals to recognize that certain foods can cause gastrointestinal distress. He was a pediatrician who suggested dietary treatment might be a benefit to some of the children with chronic diarrhea. It wasn't until 1950 that the doctoral thesis of William Dicke established that exclusion of wheat from the diet led to dramatic improvement in certain individuals suffering from recurrent diarrhea. The toxicity was shown to be a protein component, referred to as gluten. Dicke's colleagues, Weijers and Van de Kamer, showed that measurement of stool fat reflected the clinical condition. One of the ways doctors can determine if a person has severe absorption issues across the gut is if they have a high fat content in the stool. The stool will contain large amounts of fat (causing stool to float) because the gut cannot absorb it.

A true celiac cannot eat wheat, barley, or rye. There is a specific allergic reaction that occurs in the lining of the small intestines with the wheat protein called gluten. The reason a person with celiac can't eat barley or rye in addition to wheat is that their proteins are very similar to the wheat protein (Some people will also have problems with oats because its proteins are similar to wheat). This allergic reaction damages the lining of the small intestines. It can significantly affect nutrient absorption, because the small intestines are where the majority of our nutrients are absorbed into the body.

Celiac disease has the potential of affecting all aspects of the body. I cannot cover all the potential consequences of an undiagnosed celiac patient, but the initial and most common problem is not effectively absorbing food from the gut. This causes food to remain in the gut, which will result in multiple different types of gastrointestinal symptoms, such as excess gas and diarrhea. Other signs and symptoms of this disease include: liver dysfunction, with elevated liver enzymes, and heart disease. One can also have neuropsychiatric problems like depression, anxiety, and neuropathies. The bottom line is that if you suspect you have this problem, please seek out a medical evaluation by your personal physician or a gastroenterologist and have the proper testing completed to see if you have this problem.

One final piece about illness that seems caused by gluten intolerance is that there are increasing numbers of individuals who do not have true celiac disease (which can be determined by blood tests and small intestine biopsies), but seem to feel better on a gluten-free diet. These are gluten-sensitive individuals. When gluten is eliminated from their diet, they have less gastrointestinal complaints and they feel better. I have seen it clinically with my patients and a few small studies appear to corroborate that. I personally have suffered with irritable bowel symptoms all my life. I have a history of recurrent abdominal pain and bloating. I was tested and it was determined that I do not have celiac disease. However, I decided to remove gluten because of my long irritable bowel history. My symptoms have cleared up by at least 70 percent. At times when my abdominal symptoms start to reoccur, I usually find out there was something I ate earlier in the day that contained gluten.

Until recently there has been little explanation for this phenomenon. Food allergy testing has not been especially helpful. However, a book, *The Missing Microbes*, written by Dr. Martin Blaser, the former Chair of the Department of Medicine and Professor of Microbiology at New York University School of Medicine, may give us some clues as to what is going on. His explanation through years of research is that with the overuse of antibiotics, there is a loss of certain bacteria that normally inhabit the gut. Some bacteria, in particular, have been shown to down regulate our immune system. With the loss of these bacteria, through antibiotic overuse, the inability to down regulate may affect immunological reactions, such as our response to certain proteins like gluten.

The problem at this time is if you were one of the unfortunate individuals who did take a lot of antibiotics and you have this celiac-like syndrome, the only resolution at this time is to eliminate gluten. Hopefully, in the future we will be able to engineer a reintroduction of these lost bacteria to an extent that we can modify the immunologic-like effects. Unfortunately, we aren't there at this time.

By improving your digestion you can improve your overall quality of life by decreasing abdominal discomfort. This may not give you the lifesaving effects that you would receive if you prevent heart disease or cancer. However, resolving your digestive maladies can address future health issues by maximizing your absorption of food, vitamins and nutrients that are needed to maintain a healthy body.

Even though there are a few differences between what men and women eat, the two genders should generally eat the same healthy diets. The overwhelming scientific evidence shows that these diets need to be more plant based and lower in fat. Finally, unless you have a malabsorption syndrome, the usage of excessive vitamins and supplements is discouraged.

16

Weight Loss

When less is more

Over the years the majority of my patients were overweight because they made unhealthy lifestyle choices throughout their lives. The interesting fact is that most voluntarily admitted that they had made the bad choices that led to their weight gain. The good news is that if these overweight individuals decide to improve their lifestyles, the majority will lose weight.

As a physician I am concerned about individuals who are overweight, because excess weight increases the risk for multiple ailments. These risks include:

- **Brain:** strokes and dementia

- **Eyes:** cataracts

- **Lungs:** asthma, sleep apnea, and decreased ventilation syndrome

- **Heart:** high blood pressure and heart attacks

- **Liver:** fatty liver disease, with the potential of having a progressive liver disease leading to cirrhosis

- **Gallbladder:** gallstones

- **Pancreas:** pancreatitis and diabetes

- **Joints:** osteoarthritis

- **Skin:** chronic dermatitis

- **Vascular:** varicose veins

- **Cancers:** breast, esophageal, pancreatic, prostate, uterine, colorectal, and kidney

What Is Your Body Fat Percentage?

Needless to say, having a healthy weight is extremely important in disease prevention.

If you are trying to prevent these diseases, the first natural question is "What should I weigh?" A better question is, "What is my percentage of body fat?" Elevated body fat increases the risk of the above disease states. More specifically, the dreaded belly fat is the major culprit. I addressed belly fat in chapters 6 and 10 in terms of its relation to heart disease, pointing out that belly fat could produce multiple substances that can be harmful to the body. These substances can increase inflammation that not only multiplies your risk for heart disease but also can affect the body in multiple other ways, such as causing asthma and allergies.

For good general health, a man's body fat percentage should be below 25 percent (women need to be below 38 percent to be healthy). In order to be classified as fit, a man's body fat percentage needs to be less than 20 percent. Your body fat can be determined by having a health provider, a trainer, or an exercise physiologist use certain simple tools, such as fat calipers. These instruments provide a good guesstimate of your body fat. There are various other more sophisticated ways of measuring your percent of body fat. The equipment that I use at Canyon Ranch is called a dexa body scan. It is the same machine that measures bone density. This is one of the gold standards in body fat percent measurement. There are other excellent machines that are also able to measure a person's body fat. A common problem I see with fat calipers is that these tools often underestimate the actual body fat. Many times men may think they are healthy until I give them the results of their dexa scanner.

Increase Your Exercise

Generally, my first step to weight loss is not a specific diet approach; it is to get my patients moving again. This is the major difference I've seen between the genders. Women are often looking for the perfect new diet plan to help them lose weight. Men, on the other hand, are much more likely to look to exercise as their first step in weight improvement. I'm certainly not saying that women do not exercise and men don't try to diet, but my experience is that if you initially speak with a man about losing weight by changing his diet, he may turn a deaf ear to whatever you have to say. I am a perfect example of this: If my weight starts to increase, the first thing I do is look at changing my exercise program.

With most men, the road to a healthy weight begins with an exercise program. Many men need to be encouraged to begin exercising. Others need to be inspired to restart their exercise programs. Finally, there are those who need to step up and improve their existing exercise programs. Over the years I have seen that the more a person exercises, the more he tends to want to increase his exercise. This is reinforced when he starts to feel better after he has been exercising for a few weeks. Interestingly, I have noticed that once a man has started focusing on exercising, he will improve his diet next. Now the domino effect has started, and he is on the road to a better weight.

I am often asked "what is the best exercise program to lose weight?" The best exercise program is the one you can continue to do for years. It does no good to swim if you hate to swim. It's okay to experiment with different forms of exercise or to change your exercise regime seasonally. I do this every year. When spring comes along, I start to swim one to two days a week in addition to my running and cycling. When it gets cold and dark later in the fall, I usually stop swimming and start cycling more or add an extra day of running.

Of all the forms of exercise, my mainstay has always been running, because I find it so easy. I roll out of bed, put on my running gear, and step outside for a three-and-a half-mile run. It takes about thirty-five minutes, and I know it has been a good workout. I don't have to drive to a gym or pool. I need very little equipment; I just need a good pair of running shoes. To make my run more interesting, I listen to podcasts as I exercise. I get to learn something new with every run. My personal favorites are *Stuff You Should Know, The Jefferson Hour, TED Radio Hour,* and *Fresh Air* from NPR. (Listening to podcasts is not limited to when I run; I listen to podcasts when I cycle, too.) The real beauty of running is that it burns a lot of calories. Even though there are some overweight genes in my family, when I run, I never worry about my weight. Running is certainly not the best exercise for everyone—it can be tough on your knees and hips, especially if you are overweight. Find what works best for you.

Increase Your Heart Rate

Just as important as choosing an exercise program that suits you is selecting a program that is intense enough to improve your overall fitness. Walking the dog at night and stopping at every fire hydrant won't do it. Strolling through the park with your best friend or your loved one in the evenings is nice—and it is much better than sitting around watching TV—but it does not suffice when it comes to upping your fitness level. To know that you are exercising at a high enough intensity that can improve your health, you need to push your heart rate up to 70–85 percent of its maximum rate. To obtain a good estimate of your heart's maximum rate, take 220 minus your age. For example, if you are 60 years old, your estimated maximum heart rate is at 160 beats per minute (220 – 60 = 160). Then to determine the appropriate exercise intensity, take 70 percent of 160, which is 112 and 85 percent of 160, which is one 136. Therefore, at the age of 60, attaining a heart rate between 112 and 136 beats per minute during most of your exercise program means that you are now exercising effectively. You need to maintain that intensity for at least 30 minutes and perform this exercise a minimum of four to five days a week, if you want to improve your health and lose weight.

High Intensity Interval Training

If you want to improve your fitness level, or you want to burn twice as many calories during the same length of time, then consider doing high intensity interval training. This type of exercise program intermittently increases the intensity of your exercise. This intensity needs to be greater than 85 percent of your maximum heart rate (220 – age × .85). The easiest, non-mathematical way of determining if you have reached your 85 percent threshold is to increase the intensity of your chosen exercise to the point where you start to pant like a puppy dog. Increasing your intensity should be done about one quarter of the time, and you remain at that level for as long you can stand it. This will be less than two minutes; for most mortals it is less than one minute. When you slow down your exercise, return to your previous intensity of heart rate, which is between 70 and 85 percent of its maximum rate. There are multiple ways of doing this. One simple way is spending approximately 3/4 of your time in your normal aerobic pace and approximately 1/4 of the time in the high intensity state. The anaerobic portion of the exercise should be spread intermittently throughout the exercise. One way I do it is run 3/4 of a mile in a normal aerobic pace then run 1/4 of a mile at a high intense anaerobic pace. I then return back to my aerobic pace for the next 3/4 of a mile. I continue this pattern until I finish my run.

A word of caution for those of you who want to push yourselves with intermittent high-intensity exercise: It's not fun. Exercise does not necessarily have to be fun, but if you have to struggle to get out of bed to exercise in the first place, then taking part in a program that feels like it is going to kill you is certainly not encouraging you to get up. If I have a patient who has a difficult time motivating himself to exercise, I rarely encourage him to begin exercising this way. He will quit exercising shortly after starting his program. Instead, I would start him off slowly, gradually increasing the difficulty of his exercise when he's ready.

Another problem with interval training is that there is a higher risk of injuries, especially when we get older. I have personally experienced this. Almost every time I strain or pull a muscle, it is when I increase the intensity of my program. When this happens I have to stop or significantly limit my exercising for two to three months until my muscle heals.

In summary, high-intensity interval training has been shown to improve a person's fitness level. All high-level athletes use it to elevate their performance. It also has been shown to burn twice as many calories as an aerobic exercise. This is important for those individuals who have limited time to exercise or for those who have tried everything else to lose weight and have been unsuccessful.

Sugary Drinks and Obesity

Being overweight used to be a problem only with adults. Unfortunately, young men and boys are now experiencing obesity. About 40 percent of obese children have more than two risk factors for cardiovascular disease. When I first started practicing medicine 30 years ago, I never worried about high blood pressure in kids. Now, because of childhood obesity, it is a significant problem.

In looking at the dietary side of weight gain, one of the major culprits has been the beverage intake of sugary sodas and concentrated juice drinks. Forty-eight percent of the sugar consumption in this country comes from these soft drinks. In a 12-ounce soda drink, there are 10 teaspoons of sugar. Even more surprising, "healthy juice drinks" often have the same amount of sugar as the soda drinks. These concentrated calories love to pack on the pounds. We can thank all the hours of TV commercials promoting all those wonderful sweetened drinks.

If you are drinking them, stop, or the very least, significantly cut down the amount you are consuming. Many obesity experts in this country feel that one of the main causes of childhood obesity is soda drinks. I went to one of the local fast food chains and asked for a small soda, and the *small* soda was 16 ounces! The public has grown accustomed to these sweetened drinks and they want more and more. When I was in a local gas station/food mart, a customer came in and filled up a *huge* cup with soda that had at least 54 ounces in it. It looked more like a bucket with a handle on it than a drinking cup.

What about diet drinks? Even though they are supposed to have fewer calories, some studies have linked the artificial sweeteners with weight gain.[75] Other studies have revealed that diet sweeteners increase the production of insulin.[76] This excess insulin has many potential negative effects on the body that can lead to weight gain, such as increased fat deposition. Some individuals believe that artificial sweeteners condition people to want to eat more sweet foods. With the development of a "sweet tooth," a person has the tendency to eat a greater amount of sweet, calorie-dense foods, which can add on the pounds. Until this controversy is settled, I generally advise my patients to try to limit the intake of diet drinks and the use of artificial sweeteners.

Get More Sleep

A serious factor that is often overlooked in weight-loss management is the importance of sleep. This was previously discussed in the sleep chapter in relation to chronic disease. It has been shown that the prevalence of obesity was 25 percent for those individuals who averaged fewer than five hours of sleep at night.[77] One of the reasons for weight gain associated with lack of sleep is the increased production of ghrelin.[78] Ghrelin is a chemical produced in the cells that line the fundus of the stomach and epsilon cells of the pancreas. One of its major functions is to stimulate appetite. When you have a sleep deficit, your ghrelin production increases. That is why, on the days following a sleepless night, you may notice that your head is somehow sucked into the refrigerator, looking for goodies. If, after reading the chapter on sleep, you determined that you do have a sleep disturbance and you also have a weight problem, please address your sleep malady. Your ability to lose weight could become a whole lot easier.

Restrictive Dieting

One final area that I was hesitant to discuss in this chapter is some form of restrictive dieting. Before I cover this form of dieting I want it known that by far the majority of my patients can lose weight if they simply eat in a healthy way, exercise regularly, and learn to reduce stress. More than 90 percent of my patients will lose weight if they change their lifestyles. Most of my overweight patients are out of control in their lives. They are overstressed and take care of everyone but themselves. When I consider using some form of restrictive dieting, it's generally for that small minority of individuals who are doing all the right things but still can't lose weight. They have been tested for all the medical problems that can cause weight gain, such as low thyroid disease. For this small minority of frustrated overweight patients, I will consider offering some form of intermittent restrictive dieting.

Through the years I have been against the multiple different versions of restrictive dieting. One of the more recent types of restrictive dieting has been the HCG diet, which limits a person's caloric intake to 500 calories a day while he takes the hormone HCG. Other types of restrictive dieting have come in the form of liquid diets that have been promoted even within several hospital systems. People generally lose weight with restrictive eating. It doesn't take a rocket scientist to know that if you are eating very few calories, over time you will lose weight. The problem arises when a person wants to maintain that weight loss over the long term. When food is reintroduced at a more normal caloric intake, the weight tends to return. Individuals who undertake restrictive dieting look great if you see them three months after they start the diet. They often lose a ton of weight and all their friends want to know how they did it. If you don't see them again for a year, more often than not, at that next meeting they are as heavy as they were originally—and in many cases they are heavier.

While I clearly have some issues with restrictive dieting, if you remain overweight despite the fact that you are eating a good healthy diet and are exercising on a regular basis, you may want to consider a modified version of restrictive eating. What do we know about restrictive dieting? I recommend reading *The Fast Diet* by Dr. Michael Mosley of England, an excellent book that looks at the scientific evidence on forms of restrictive dieting. He examined the research from Dr. Longo of the University of Southern California's longevity center and Dr. Mark Mattson of the National Institute of Aging. Through their research (unfortunately, mostly with rats) they have shown that some forms of restrictive eating can cause:

- Weight loss

- Increased longevity

- Switching on repair genes. When we have all the food we can eat, our bodies are designed to grow and have sex. During fasting, the body believes it is entering a famine state. Since the genes for growth and sex are placed on hold, the body senses it's a good time to repair.

- Decreased levels of IGF-1. This hormone has growth effects. There have been implications of increased IGF-1 and cancer growth.

- With intermittent fasting, insulin levels decrease and there is increased insulin sensitivity (Elevated levels of insulin are associated with increased fat storage and increased appetite).

- With fasting mice there is an increased production of BDNF (brain derived neurotrophic factor). BDNF has been shown to stimulate stem cells to turn into new nerve cells in the area of the brain called your hippocampus, which is essential in memory.

- There are indications (with the rats) that it may delay the onset of dementia.

Dr. Mosley's work clearly illustrates that fasting seems to have beneficial effects. The problem has always been one of sustainability. There are multiple ways to intermittently restrict your diet. When most people think of fasting, they have visions of Gandhi not eating for days on end. This is not what Dr. Mosley and others have promoted. Intermittent or very controlled eating appears to have some of the same effects. Dr. Mosley promotes the 5/2 diet, in which five days a week a person eats a regular healthy diet, and two non-contiguous days during that week he advises eating 600 calories (for women it is 500 calories). Dr. Longo's version is that he himself skips lunch every day.

I personally was interested in this and decided to delay my intake of breakfast. This is against everything I have preached over the years. My first concern was that I would have a rebound increased caloric intake with my lunch. That did not occur (other studies have also shown this). In fact, I lost five pounds over a two-week period, and I really wasn't particularly overweight from the onset. I started at 178 pounds and dropped to 173 pounds. Since doing this I have maintained my weight loss, and my overall energy level is as good as it has been in years.

The bottom line is that a modified form of restrictive dieting may be for you if you have tried multiple weight-loss programs and have been unsuccessful. Lastly, it should go without saying that whenever you do eat, make sure your choices are healthy ones.

Weight loss is not just a means of trying to look better. It is important in the prevention of multiple disease states. More often than not a man will get to an unhealthy overweight state by simply overeating, not exercising, and being overstressed. The answer to weight loss may be just as simple. Don't overeat—especially overly sugary foods. Perform regular exercise that have some degree of intensity, and learn ways to deal with undue stress.

Epigenetics

We can help our genes.

The basic facts of life are that if you exercise regularly, eat a healthy, well-balanced diet with lots of fruits and vegetables, and do the best you can to manage stress odds are you will live a long healthy life. Our environment can have a major influence on our genes. I personally have had my whole DNA genome sequenced, and according to what my genes say, I should have left this planet years ago. So how am I here writing this book, still running three miles a day, and planning on working another twenty years? How is this possible? The answer is epigenetics. This field of science is relatively new. We have known for years that people who make wise, healthy choices tend to live longer, healthier lives. Sure it improves our blood sugars and our cholesterol levels, but it does more than that. It can affect our genes. Healthy lifestyles can essentially turn genes on or off in a positive way, and poor lifestyles can also turn genes on and off in a negative way.

You Can Change Your Genes with Your Choices

On top of a person's DNA (that's why it is called epigenetics) are biochemical marks (some call them tags). These marks are capable of modulating DNA activity and functions but do not alter the DNA sequence. The marks are dynamic and not fixed. They are strongly influenced by the environment and exposure to external factors, including diet, living conditions, exercise, stress, chemicals, drugs, and toxins. In the broad sense it is a link between a person's genetic makeup and his actual physical appearance or expression.

These epigenetic marks work by regulating gene activity. You may have the gene to develop premature heart disease, but by making the right healthy choices you may be able to produce an epigenetic mark that will actually turn off that gene. This is why I get up out of bed at 5:00 a.m. and run! These epigenetic marks operate by activating or inactivating genes through altering the amount of protein that is synthesized or expressed by a gene. It can also determine when a gene is expressed throughout the course of a lifetime. There are at least three different mechanisms that can accomplish this. The first and most studied is methylation. A methyl group, which is CH3, binds to cytosine, which is one of the four-nucleotide bases of DNA (the others are guanine, adenine, and thymine). When the methyl group binds to cytosine, it has the capability of silencing or turning off that gene.

The second way our bodies can modify gene expression involves modification of histone proteins. These proteins help organize DNA structure. DNA wraps around these histone proteins like beads on a necklace. The tighter the DNA wraps around the proteins, the less exposure the genes have to be expressed because of the inability of messenger RNA to access the genes. The reverse is true in that as the DNA loosens up its attachment to the histone protein, the better the access messenger RNA has to the gene. This increases the likelihood of expressing the genes. A simple way of looking at these two epigenetic effects is to think of your genes as some type of electrical devise where methylation is the switch to turn that equipment on or off and the histone modification is the knob that turns the volume of that equipment up or down.

A third type of epigenetic effect is with non-coding RNA. This particular RNA can target specific messenger RNA and simply prevent their translation to make certain proteins.

This ability to effect a gene's expression was recently shown through a study performed by Dean Ornish, MD, and fellow researchers. They looked at a group of men with low-grade prostate cancer, who decided to do active surveillance (see page 130). These men adopted a low-fat, plant-based diet, started on a regular exercise program, and practiced stress management by attending group support sessions. Gene expression profiles were obtained from the participants, pairing RNA samples from control prostate needle biopsy taken before intervention to RNA from the same patient's 3-month postintervention biopsy. Quantitative real-time PCR was used to validate array observations for selected transcripts. Two-class paired analysis of global gene expression using significance analysis of microarrays detected 48 up-regulated (turned on) and 453 (turned off) down-regulated transcripts after the intervention.[79] This pilot study has shown how improving lifestyles can modulate the expression of genes in the prostate.

Other work that has shown the ability to effect gene expression was demonstrated to me by Travis Dunckley, PhD, from Translational Genomics Research Institute (better know as TGen). He presented one of the more remarkable lectures I have seen in years at Canyon Ranch. He showed us photographs of DNA microarrays. This is a remarkable colored picture (made by marking methylated areas of DNA with a florescent dye) that scientists use to illustrate the degree of methylation in a person's genes. Dr. Dunckley presented a composite microarray of individuals eating a plant-based diet versus a microarray composite of individuals eating a typical Western diet full of red meat, fats, few fruits and vegetables, and plenty of concentrated carbohydrates. They looked entirely different. It was day and night. Nothing has shown me more about how our environment can have such a huge effect on our gene expression than these microarray photos.

≈≈≈

One final note on this subject is that epigenetic activity was originally thought to be one generational. This is not the case. It has been shown that these epigenetic marks can potentially be trans-generational. Therefore, we actually may pay for the sins of our parents. If our parents engaged in unhealthy activities, especially when we were in utero (in Mom's belly), it could have a negative effect on us. For example, there is evidence in the Norwegian Mother and Child Birth Cohort[80] that revealed that the mothers who smoked during their pregnancy had changes in methylation of their offspring. Hopefully, by bathing ourselves in a healthy environment, we can turn off the genes that were initially turned on by the bad habits of our parents and turn on those genes that can keep us healthy.

18

Meditation Works

Give it a try.

When I grew up in the 60s, the practice of meditation was first being noticed by the general public in the Western world. Much of this movement began when the Beatles returned from India with their ideas of Transcendental Meditation. It wasn't until I started working at Canyon Ranch that I personally considered the practice of meditation. I was amazed at the number of my co-workers and patients who were meditating regularly. Before I considered the actual practice of meditation for myself, I wanted to approach meditation with an open mind, so I decided to look into the actual science of meditation. As I read the literature, I found out that the actual practice of meditation has been going on for thousands of years. It began in India with the Vedas and Buddhists. It has been used in almost every religion, but it is not a religious experience.

My Path to Meditation

After reading several scientific articles on meditation, I decided it was time to experience it for myself. I didn't have to go very far to accomplish this task. I simply stepped out of my medical office and walked across the courtyard to the department of behavioral health. I asked their receptionist if any of the therapists had time to talk to me, and she said that John Shukwit was available. That was fortunate because John is a known expert in meditation. I walked down the hall and when I reached John's office, he wanted to know what special occasion had brought the medical director over to his side of the courtyard. I told him I was there to learn how to practice meditation, but I was in a hurry and had to be back in my office in ten minutes. John smiled but politely declined my request, because he said there was really no way he could teach me how to meditate in only ten minutes. I thought that was ridiculous. How hard could it be to close your eyes, cross your legs, and repeat some phrase? I told him in the time it had taken him to tell me he couldn't teach me how to meditate he was now down to eight minutes.

Because I had always ignored John's sessions on meditation in the past, he realized that this might be the only chance he had to introduce me to this ancient practice. He finally relented and asked me to sit and relax in the chair. At that point he had me close my eyes and in my mind count to six on my inspiration, hold my breath for a count of two, and then count to six during my expiration. He then had me repeat this sequence many times. After what felt to be a very long time, John told me that my time was up and that I could return to the medical department. When I got up from my chair, I thanked him for his time, but in the back of my mind I thought, *how in the world could closing your eyes and counting actually have any real effect on a person's health?*

As I walked back across the courtyard to the medical building I decided to stop in our employee dining area to get something to drink. When I walked in, one of our medical receptionists was watching TV. I did not say a word to her, but she suddenly stopped watching the TV, looked at me for a few seconds, and said out of nowhere,

"What's wrong with you? Why are you so calm?" I could not believe what she said. My less than ten-minute impromptu meditative session had produced a noticeable relaxation change to this skeptic. Nothing changed my opinion more on what meditation was capable of doing than that little exchange in the employee-dining lounge.

It was still hard for me to accept that sitting with your legs crossed (don't worry, you don't actually have to cross your legs), closing your eyes, and doing some deep slow breathing could actually make a real difference in a person's health. Even with my positive eight-minute meditation session, I was having a difficult time believing that meditation could make a person healthier. I decided to look further into recent scientific studies related to meditation. To my surprise the evidence is pretty clear that the simple exercise of meditation has a positive effect on a person's health.

The Benefits of Meditation

Meditation can lower a person's overall level of stress.[81] Chronic stress is a known contributing factor in multiple disease states. One of those diseases is atherosclerosis (hardening of the arteries). Chronic stress can cause platelet dysfunction, which affects blood clotting. Stress can injure the lining of the arterial walls (this is called endothelial dysfunction) by causing the production of excess stimulants, such as adrenalin. These stimulants can then damage arteries by causing them to go into spasms and subsequently elevating blood pressure. Regular practice of meditation has also been shown to impact the negative cardiovascular effects of stress by decreasing a person's blood pressure.[82]

Meditation can have a positive effect on our endocrine system. It has been shown to lower cortisol levels.[83] Prolonged elevations of cortisol can lead to increased blood sugars and potentially the development of diabetes.

In addition to decreasing the risk of developing heart disease and diabetes, daily meditation appears to have a positive effect on the brain. The size of the brain has been shown to increase with meditation. There have studies that have actually shown that meditation can increase the size of the brain.[84] As I get older, anything I can do that has the potential of increasing my brain size has a huge appeal to me. Meditation can also positively affect the brain by increasing its blood flow.[85] In the study cited, it revealed that cerebral blood flow increased in the frontal and occipital brain regions in the meditating group compared to the control group. This effect appears to be related to a decreased cerebrovascular resistance (the blood vessels dilate) during meditation.

Besides decreasing stress and anxiety, meditation has been found to be effective against depression.[86] Medications have been the mainstay of therapy for those individuals who suffer from moderate to severe depression. Anyone who has been on an antidepressant knows that these medications can be helpful in pulling a person out of the depths of depression and in many ways they can be lifesaving. The unfortunate aspect of many antidepressants, especially if more than one medication needs to be used, is the potential for developing side effects. Some of those side effects were discussed in the sexual function chapter; this included decreased libido and erectile dysfunction. Since the scientific evidence for treating depression with routine meditation practice is well documented in the literature,[87] I have recommended it for my depressed patients. With meditation I have been able to decrease the dose of the patient's antidepressants, lower the number of antidepressants, or in some cases actually eliminate them altogether.

Types of Meditation

There are basically three forms of meditation: focused attention meditation, mindfulness meditation, and compassion meditation.[88]

Focused meditation is the one I usually recommend to my patients and the form I personally practice. This type of meditation is a way of calming the mind. In our hectic lives we are often thinking of twenty different things; we worry about what went wrong yesterday and fret about everything that we must deal with tomorrow. This pattern leads to anxiety and stress. The simple way to attain a focused meditative state is to find a quiet space and sit comfortably in a chair or on the floor. Do whatever is comfortable for you. Close your eyes and either take slow rhythmic breaths, focusing on your inspiration and expiration, or you count slowly with an inspiration to an arbitrary number like five or six, hold your breath for a two or three counts, then expire your air while counting in your head to five or six. For example, counting sheep is a type of focused meditation to help quiet your mind so that you can fall asleep.

You can go to: https://www.facebook.com/TheCanyonRanch GuidetoMensHealth/ and view a short video on focused meditation by my daughter, Elizabeth, who is a yoga and meditation teacher at Canyon Ranch.

The second form of meditation is called mindfulness. The meditator becomes aware of his surroundings without developing attachments to them. You can take note of everything without being overly preoccupied with any one specific object. Over time this detached perspective can allow you to be less annoyed by many of those little things that often seem to grind us. This, in time, can lower your overall anxiety and stress levels.

The third type of meditation is compassionate meditation. The objective of this type of meditation is to have concern for those who suffer. This means that a person will give support and care for those who suffer but will not fall into the potentially destructive empathetic path of caring. If someone is overly empathetic, he can become entwined in the pain of the one who is suffering. A person often pays a price for doing this, and it can wear him down and can cause burn-out. This is seen in caregivers who become overly attached to their patients or teachers who get over-involved with their students. Not only can it negatively affect the caregiver but also it can be detrimental to the person who is suffering. A person who performs compassionate meditation is present, helpful, and more objective for those who suffer. Who would you rather care for you if you were sick, someone fretting and pacing about the room or someone who is calm and present with you at your side?

~~~~

Is meditation the Holy Grail of health? The quick answer to that question is no. However, unlike exercise, which takes work and effort to complete, there is little effort involved. So, yes, many men do meditate. This powerful tool should be considered a part of everyone's daily lives to improve their overall health.

Epilogue

My objective in writing this book was to encourage men to take a better look at their health and to give my best advice on how to improve it at each phase of our lives. The future is much brighter and more fun if you proceed through life in a healthy state. Spending time trying to catch up, or unable to participate in activities with our kids or grandkids, can be extremely frustrating.

I hope that after reading this book and embodying the advice and directions given, you will not only keep up with others but also be a leader in your family or group. I have seen this in my personal life. My 24-year-old daughter, a fitness expert and yoga-instructor, is so proud of my healthy lifestyle and resultant good health that she likes to invite me to meet her friends. She loves to tell them I am actually a young man in my sixties. What more could a dad ask for!

Endnotes

1. National Center for Health Statistics, *Health, United States, 2013: With Special Feature on Prescription Drugs.* Accessed September 2, 2015. http://www.cdc.gov/nchs/data/hus/hus13.pdf#015.

2. Centers for Disease Control and Prevention, *Mortality Tables.* Accessed September 2, 2015. http://www.cdc.gov/men/lcod/2009/LCOD_menal-lages2009.pdf.

3. James R. Couch and Candace Bearss, "Headache in the Post-trauma Syndrome: Relation to Extent of Head Injury," *Headache* 41:6 (2001): 559–564. http://www.ncbi.nlm.nih.gov/pubmed/11437891#.

4. C. W. Hoge, et al., "Mild Traumatic Brain Injury in US Soldiers Returning from Iraq," *New England Journal of Medicine* 358:5 (2008): 453. doi: 10.1056/NEJMoa072972.

5. C. W. Wu, et al., "Hypothalamic-Pituitary-Testicular Axis Disruptions in Older Men Are Differentially Linked to Age and Modifiable Risk Factors: The European Male Aging Study," *Journal of Clinical Endocrinology and Metabolism* 93:7 (2008): 2737–2745. doi: 10.1210/jc.2007-1972.

6. Francesco Sofi, et al., "Adherence to Mediterranean Diet and Health Status: Meta-analysis," *British Medical Journal* 337 (2008): a1344. doi: 10.1136/bmj.a1344.

7. National Institute of Health of the National Academy of Sciences, *Review of the Health Effects in Vietnam Veterans of Exposure to Herbicides,* 9th Biennial Update. Accessed Sept. 2, 2015. http://iom.nationalacademies.org/Activities/Veterans/AgentOrangeNinthUpdate.aspx

8. William Glaberson, "Agent Orange, the Next Generation," *The New York Times,* August 8, 2004. http://www.nytimes.com/2004/08/08/nyregion/08orange.html.

9. *Review of the Health Effects in Vietnam Veterans.*

10. *Review of the Health Effects in Vietnam Veterans.*

11. Harvard Men's Health Watch, "Is Sex Exercise? And is it Hard on the Heart?" *Harvard Health Publications* (June 2011). Accessed September 2, 2015. http://www.health.harvard.edu/newsletter_article/is-sex-exercise-and-is-it-hard-on-the-heart.

12. Susan A. Hall, et al., "Sexual Activity, Erectile Dysfunction, and Incident Cardiovascular Events," *American Journal of Cardiology* 105:2 (2010): 192–197. doi: 10.1016/j.amjcard.2009.08.671.

13. S. J. Berry, et al., "The Development of Human Benign Prostatic Hyperplasia with Age," *Journal of Urology* 132:3 (1984: 474–479). http://www.ncbi.nlm.nih.gov/pubmed/6206240.

14. U. Schwarzer, et al., "The Prevalence of Peyronie's Disease: Results of a Large Survey," *BJU International* 88:7 (2001): 727–30. doi: 10.1046/j.1464-4096.2001.02436.

15. William D. Finkle, et al., "Increased Risk of Non-fatal Myocardial Infarction Following Testosterone Therapy Prescription in Men," *PloS one* 9:1 (2014): e85805. doi: 10.1371/journal.pone.0085805.

16. J. Baillargeon J, et al., "Risk of Myocardial Infarction in Older Men Receiving Testosterone Therapy," *The Annals of Pharmacotherapy* 48:9 (2014):1138–1144. doi: 10.1177/1060028014539918.

17. S. Basaria, et al., "Effects of Testosterone Administration for 3 Years on Subclinical Atherosclerosis Progression in Older Men with Low or Low-Normal Testosterone Levels: A Randomized Clinical Trial," *JAMA* 314:6 (2015): 570–581. doi: 10.1001/jama.2015.8881.

18. M. Falb, A. Figueroa, and D. Kanny, *2006 Georgia School Health Profiles Report* (Georgia Department of Human Resources: 2007). Accessed September 2, 2015. http://dph.georgia.gov/sites/dph.georgia.gov/files/2006_School_Health_Profiles_FINAL.pdf.

19. Sherry L. Murphy, et al., "Deaths Final data for 2010," *National Vital Statistics Reports* 61: 4 (Hyattsville, MD: National Center for Health Statistics, 2013).

20. "Heart Disease Mortality Data Trends for 2000-2008: Race/Ethnic Group Differences," California Department of Public Health. Accessed September 2, 2015. http://www.cdph.ca.gov/programs/ohir/Pages/Heart2008Race.aspx.

21. "Who is at Risk for Coronary Heart Disease?" National Heart, Lung and Blood Institute. Last updated September 29, 2014. Accessed September 2, 2015. http://www.nhlbi.nih.gov/health/health-topics/topics/cad/atrisk.html

22. "Who is at Risk for Coronary Heart Disease?"

23. Paul A. James, et al., "2014 Evidence-Based Guideline for the Management of High Blood Pressure in Adults Report From the Panel Members Appointed to the Eighth Joint National Committee (JNC 8)," *JAMA* 311: 5 (2014): 507–520. doi: 10.1001/jama.2013.284427.

24. "Who is at Risk for Coronary Heart Disease?"

25. Timo A. Lakka, et al., "Effects of Exercise Training on Plasma Levels of C-Reactive Protein in Healthy Subjects: the HERITAGE Family Study," *European Heart Journal* 26:19 (2005): 2018–2025. doi: http://dx.doi.org/10.1093/eurheartj/ehi394.

26. Taulant Muka, et al., "Polyunsaturated Fatty Acids and Serum C-reactive Protein: the Rotterdam Study," *American Journal of Epidemiology* 181:11 (2015): 846–856. doi: 10.1093/aje/kwv021.

27. "Who is at Risk for Coronary Heart Disease?"

28. Goran Walldius, et al., "High Apolipoprotein B, Low Apolipoprotein A-I, and Improvement in the Prediction of Fatal Myocardial Infarction: A Prospective Study," *Lancet* 358:9298 (2001): 2026–2033. doi: http://dx.doi.org/10.1016/S0140-6736(01)07098-2.

29. Frank B. Hu, et al., "Dietary Fat Intake and the Risk of Coronary Heart Disease in Women," *New England Journal of Medicine* 337:21 (1997):1491–9. doi: 10.1056/NEJM199711203372102.

30. Benoît Lamarche, et al., "Fasting Insulin and Apolipoprotein B Levels and Low-Density Lipoprotein Particle Size as Risk Factors for Ischemic Heart Disease," *JAMA* 279:24 (1998): 1955–1961. doi:10.1001/jama.279.24.1955.

31. "FDA to Extend Comment Period on Measure to Further Reduce Trans Fat in Processed Foods—Update," www.fda.gov. Last updated December 30, 2013. Accessed September 2, 2015. http://www.fda.gov/Food/NewsEvents/ConstituentUpdates/ucm379916.htm

32. Iris Shai, et al., "Lipoprotein (a) and Coronary Heart Disease among Women: Beyond a Cholesterol Carrier?" *European Heart Journal* 26:16 (2005): 1633–1639. doi: http://dx.doi.org/10.1093/eurheartj/ehi222.

33. Folgerdiena M. de Vries, Kolthof J1, Postma MJ1, Denig P2, Hak E1 "Efficacy of Standard and Intensive Statin Treatment for the Secondary Prevention of Cardiovascular and Cerebrovascular Events in Diabetes Patients: A Meta-analysis," *PLoS one* 9:11 (2014): e111247. doi: 10.1371/journal.pone.0111247.

34. Marc S. Penn and Andrea B. Klemes, "Multimarker Approach for Identifying and Documenting Mitigation of Cardiovascular Risk," *Future Cardiology* 9:4 (2013): 497–506. doi: 10.2217/fca.13.27.

35. J. L. Cracowski, et al., "Increased Formation of F2-Isoprostanes in Patients with Severe Heart Failure," *Heart* 84:4 (2000): 439–440. doi:10.1136/heart.84.4.439.

36. Paul Holvoet, et al., "Circulating Oxidized LDL is a Useful Marker for Identifying Patients with Coronary Artery disease," *Arteriosclerosis, Thrombosis, and Vascular Biology* 21 (2001): 844–848. doi: 10.1161/01.ATV.21.5.844.

37. John S. Yudkin, Richard D. Forrest, and Caroline A. Jackson, "Microalbuminuria as Predictor of Vascular Disease in Non-Diabetic Subjects," *Lancet* 332:8610 (1988): 530–533. doi: http://dx.doi.org/10.1016/S0140-6736(88)92657-8.

38. Nisha Dada, Nam W. Kim, and Robert L. Wolfert, "Lp-PLA2: An Emerging Biomarker of Coronary Heart Disease," *Expert Review of Molecular Diagnostics* 2:1 (2002): 17–22. doi:10.1586/14737159.2.1.17.

39. Renliang Zhang, et al., "Association Between Myeloperoxidase Levels and Risk of Coronary Artery Disease," *JAMA* 286:17 (2001): 2136–2142. doi:10.1001/jama.286.17.2136.

40. Alice S. Whittemore, et al ., "Family History and Prostate Cancer Risk in Black, White, and Asian Men in United States and Canada," *American Journal of Epidemiology* 141:8 (1995): 732–740. http://www.ncbi.nlm.nih.gov/pubmed/7535977.

41. Maurice P. A. Zeegers, Annemarie Jellema, and Harry Ostrer, "Empiric Risk of Prostate Carcinoma for Relatives of Patients with Prostate Carcinoma: A Meta-analysis," *Cancer* 97:8 (2003):1894–1903. doi: 10.1002/cncr.11262.

42. Deborah Thompson, Douglas F. Easton, and the Breast Cancer Linkage Consortium, "Cancer Incidence in BRCA1 Mutation Carriers," *Journal of the National Cancer Institute* 94:18 (2002):1358–1365. doi: 10.1093/jnci/94.18.1358.

43. Breast Cancer Linkage Consortium, "Cancer Risks in BRCA2 Mutation Carriers," *Journal of the National Cancer Institute* 91:15 (1999):1310–1316. doi: 10.1093/jnci/91.15.1310.

44. Ian M. Thompson, et al., "The Influence of Finasteride on the Development of Prostate Cancer," *New England Journal of Medicine* 349:3 (2003): 215. doi: 10.1056/NEJMoa030660.

45. William J. Catalona, et al., "Comparison of Digital Rectal Examination and Serum Prostate Specific Antigen in the Early Detection of Prostate Cancer: Results of a Multicenter Clinical Trial of 6,630 Men," *Journal of Urology* 151:5 (1994):1283. http://www.ncbi.nlm.nih.gov/pubmed/7512659.

46. D. S. Smith, William J. Catalona, "Rate of Change in Serum Prostate Specific Antigen Levels as a Method for Prostate Cancer Detection," *Journal of Urology* 152:4 (1994):116. http://www.ncbi.nlm.nih.gov/pubmed/7520949.

47. Joanne Frattaroli, et al., "Clinical Events in Prostate Cancer Lifestyle Trial: Results from Two Years of Follow-Up," *Urology* 72:6 (2008): 1319–23. doi: 10.1016/j.urology.2008.04.050.

48. Teodoro del Ser, et al., "Cognitive Deficiency in Mild Hypothyroidism," *Neurologia* 15:5 (2000):193. http://www.ncbi.nlm.nih.gov/pubmed/10850118.

49. Daniel P. Perl MD, "Neuropathology of Alzheimer's Disease," *Mount Sinai Journal of Medicine* 77:1 (2010): 32–42. doi: 10.1002/msj.20157.

50. Alzheimer's Association, "2012 Alzheimer's Disease Facts and Figures," *Alzheimer's & Dementia* 8:2 (212): 131–168. doi: 10.1016/j.jalz.2012.02.001.

51. Sudha Seshadri, et al., "The Lifetime Risk of Stroke: Estimates from the Framingham Study," *Stroke* 37:2 (2006):345–50. doi: 10.1161/01.STR.0000199613.38911.b2.

52. Friedrich H. Lewy, "Paralysis agitans" in *Handbuch der Neurologie*, ed. M. Lawandowsky (Berlin: Springer-Verlag, 1912), 920.

53. Joe Verghese, et al., "Leisure Activities and the Risk of Dementia in the Elderly," *New England Journal of Medicine* 348:2508 (2003): 2516. doi: 10.1056/NEJMoa022252.

54. Stanley J. Colcombe, et al., "Aerobic Exercise Training Increases Brain Volume in Aging Humans." *The Journals of Gerontology, Series A* 61:11 (2006): 1166–1170. http://www.ncbi.nlm.nih.gov/pubmed/17167157.

55. Domenico Praticò, et al., "Increase of Brain Oxidative Stress in Mild Cognitive Impairment: A Possible Predictor of Alzheimer Disease," *JAMA Neurology* 59:6 (2002): 972–976. doi:10.1001/archneur.59.6.972.

56. Shirley Zafra-Stone, et al., "Berry Anthocyanins as Novel Antioxidants in Human Health and Disease Prevention," *Molecular Nutrition and Food Research* 51:6 (2007): 675–683. doi: 10.1002/mnfr.200700002.

57. Marjo H. Eskelinen and Miia Kivipelto, "Caffeine as a Protective Factor in Dementia and Alzheimer's Disease," *Journal of Alzheimer's Disease* 20:S1 (2010): 167–174. doi: 10.3233/JAD-2010-1404.

58. Rafal Marciniak, et al., "Effect of Meditation on Cognitive Functions in Context of Aging and Neurodegenerative Diseases," *Frontiers in Behavioral Neurosciences* 8 (2014): 17. doi: 10.3389/fnbeh.2014.00017.

59. Patrick Dale, "Examples of Isotonic & Isometric Exercises." Livestrong.com. Last updated December 18, 2013. Accessed September 3, 2015. http://www.livestrong.com/article/373853-examples-of-isotonic-isometric-exercises/.

60. Michelle Matte, "Isotonic vs. Isometric Muscle Exercises." Livestrong.com. Last updated January 28, 2015. Accessed September 3, 2015. http://www.livestrong.com/article/449913-isotonic-vs-isometric-muscle-exercises/.

61. Justin C. Brown and Kathryn H. Schmitz, "Weight Lifting and Physical Function Among Survivors of Breast Cancer: A Post Hoc Analysis of a Randomized Controlled Trial," *Journal of Clinical Oncology* 33:19 (2015): 2184–9. doi: 10.1200/JCO.2014.57.7395.

62. Teresa Opdycke, "Stretching Your Way To Flexibility: Learn Basic Stretching Techniques And Benefits." lifescript.com. Last updated September 21, 2007. Accessed September 3, 2015. http://www.lifescript.com/diet-fitness/articles/s/stretching_your_way_to_flexibility.aspx.

63. Karoline Cheung, Patria A. Hume, and Linda Maxwell, "Delayed Onset Muscle Soreness," *Sports Medicine* 33:2 (2003): 145–164. http://www.ncbi.nlm.nih.gov/pubmed/12617692.

64. Murray W Johns, "A New Method for Measuring Daytime Sleepiness: The Epworth Sleepiness Scale," *Sleep* 14:6 (1991): 540–545.

65. Meeta Singh, et al., "The Association Between Obesity and Short Sleep Duration: A Population-Based Study," *Journal of Clinical Sleep Medicine* 1:4 (2005): 357–63. http://www.ncbi.nlm.nih.gov/pubmed/17564401.

66. Jane Wardle, et al., "Gender Differences in Food Choice: The Contribution of Health Beliefs and Dieting," *Annals of Behavioral Medicine* 27:2 (2004): 107–116. http://www.ncbi.nlm.nih.gov/pubmed/15053018.

67. An Pan, et al., "Red Meat Consumption and Mortality: Results from 2 Prospective Cohort Studies," *Archives of Internal Medicine* 172:7 (2012): 555–563. doi: 10.1001/archinternmed.2011.2287.

68. Robert A. Koeth, et al., "Intestinal Microbiota Metabolism of L-Carnitine, a Nutrient in Red Meat, Promotes Atherosclerosis," *Nature Medicine* 19:5 (2013): 576–85. doi: 10.1038/nm.3145.

69. Xiang Gao, Michael P. LaValley, and Katherine L. Tucker, "Prospective Studies of Dairy Product and Calcium Intakes and Prostate Cancer Risk: A Meta-Analysis," *Journal of the National Cancer Institute* 97:23 (2005):1768.

70. Dean Ornish, et al., "Intensive Lifestyle Changes for Reversal of Coronary Heart Disease," *JAMA* 280:23 (1998): 2001–2007. doi:10.1001/jama.280.23.2001.

71. Gao, LaValley, Tucker, "Prospective Studies of Dairy Product and Calcium Intakes."

72. J. J. DiNicolantonio, et al., "Omega-3s and Cardiovascular Health," *The Ochsner Journal* 14:3 (2014): 399–412. http://www.ncbi.nlm.nih.gov/pubmed/25249807.

73. Theodore M. Brasky, et al., "Plasma Phospholipid Fatty Acids and Prostate Cancer Risk in the SELECT Trial," *Journal of the National Cancer Institute* 105:15 (2013): 1132–1141. doi: 10.1093/jnci/djt174.

74. Laura E. Targownik, et al., "Use of Proton Pump Inhibitors and Risk of Osteoporosis-Related Fractures," *Canadian Medical Association Journal* 179:4 (2008): 319–326. doi: 10.1503/cmaj.071330.

75. Susan E. Swithers and Terry L. Davidson, "A Role for Sweet Taste: Calorie Predictive Relations in Energy Regulation by Rats," *Behavioral Neuroscience* 122:1 (2008): 161–173. doi: 10.1037/0735-7044.

76. M. Yanina Pepino, et al., "Sucralose Affects Glycemic and Hormonal Responses to an Oral Glucose Load," *Diabetes Care* 36:9 (2013): 2530–2535. doi: 10.2337/dc12-2221.

77. Meeta Singh, et al., "The Association Between Obesity and Short Sleep Duration."

78. Karine Spiegel, et al., "Brief Communication: Sleep Curtailment in Healthy Young Men is Associated with Decreased Leptin Levels, Elevated Ghrelin Level, and Increase Hunger and Appetite," *Annals of Internal Medicine* 141:11 (2004): 846–850. doi:10.7326/0003-4819-141-11-200412070-00008.

79. Dean Ornish, et al., "Changes in Prostate Gene Expression in Men Undergoing an Intensive Nutrition and Lifestyle Intervention," *Proceedings of the National Academy of Sciences* 105:24 (2008): 8369–8374. doi: 10.1073/pnas.0803080105.

80. "Norwegian Mother and Child Birth Cohort." Norwegian Institute of Public Health. Accessed September 3, 2015. http://www.fhi.no/eway/default.

81. Claudia Carrisoli, Daniela Villani, and Giuseppe Riva, "Does a Meditation Protocol Supported by a Mobile Application Help People Reduce Stress? Suggestions from a Controlled Pragmatic Trial," *Cyberpsychology, Behavior and Social Networking* 18:1 (2015): 46–53. doi: 10.1089/cyber.2014.0062.

82. Sergei Pavlov, et al., "Impact of Long-Term Meditation Practice on Cardiovascular Reactivity During Perception and Reappraisal of Affective Images," *International Journal of Psychophysiology* 95:3 (2015): 363–371. doi: 10.1016/j.ijpsycho.2015.01.002.

83. Francesco Bottaccioli, et al., "Brief Training of Psychoneuroendocrinoimmunology-based Meditation (PNEIMED) Reduces Stress Symptom Ratings and Improves Control on Salivary Cortisol Secretion Under Basal and Stimulated Conditions," *Explore (NY)* 10:3 (2014): 170–9. doi: 10.1016/j.explore.2014.02.002.

84. Florian Krutch, et al., "Brain Gray Matter Changes Associated with Mindfulness Meditation in Older Adults: An Exploratory Pilot Study using Voxel-based Morphometry." *Neuro: Open Journal* 1:1 (2014): 23–26.

85. R. Jevning, et al., "Effects on Regional Cerebral Blood Flow of Transcendental Meditation," *Physiology & Behavior* 59:3 (1996): 399–402. doi:10.1016/0031-9384(95)02006-3.

86. Felipe A. Jain, et al., "Critical Analysis of the Efficacy of Meditation Therapies for Acute and Subacute Phase Treatment of Depressive Disorders: A Systematic Review," *Psychosomatics* 56:2 (2014): 140–152. doi: 10.1016/j.psym.2014.10.007.

87. M. H. Delui, et al., "Comparison of Cardiac Rehabilitation Programs Combined with Relaxation and Meditation Techniques on Reduction of Depression and Anxiety of Cardiovascular Patients," *Open Cardiovascular Medicine Journal* 7 (2013): 99–103. doi: 10.2174/1874192401307010099.

88. Matthieu Ricard, Antoine Lutz, and Richard J. Davidson, "Mind of the Mediator," *Scientific American* 311:5 (2014): 38–45. doi:10.1038/scientificamerican1114-38

Index

T

About the Author

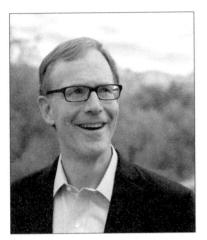

Stephen Brewer, MD, is a board certified family physician. He received his BS from The Ohio State University, graduated from medical school at the Medical College of Ohio, and completed his family medicine residency at Riverside Methodist Hospital in Columbus, Ohio. Under the direction of Andrew Weil, MD, he later completed a fellowship in integrative medicine at the University of Arizona. He is also certified in medical acupuncture and guided imagery.

Dr. Brewer began his medical career as a country doctor in the small Midwestern town where he was born and raised. He returned to Riverside Methodist Hospital to serve as Assistant Director of Family Medicine. From RMH, he moved to Cincinnati, Ohio and started Madeira Family Practice, which, over the course of seventeen years, he established as one of the largest private family practices in the area. During his last four years there, he simultaneously served as the first medical director of Integrative Medicine for the TriHealth Hospital system.

Since 2004, Dr. Brewer has been Medical Director at Canyon Ranch in Tucson, Arizona. He consults with patients regarding complex diagnoses, preventive care, executive health, and men's health. He provides lectures to specialized audiences on the aforementioned concerns, as well as brain health, cardiovascular health, weight loss, integrative medicine, and peak performance. He serves as Canyon Ranch's liaison with Mayo Clinic and the University of Arizona.

Dr. Brewer is an internationally featured speaker. His credits include appearances on *The Dr. Oz Radio Show*, the *Today Show*, and CNN. He coauthored *The Everest Principle: How to Achieve the Summit of Your Life* (2010). His web credits include Maria Shriver's Women's Conference, "The Everest Principle or How to Reach Your Peak Performance"; Oprah.com "Peak Performance"; and Active.com "Acupuncture for Athletes" and "Peak Performance and Sleep." He has been published in the *Ohio Academy of Family Practice News* medical journal.